Intermittent Fasting

An Exhaustive Guide For Novices On Efficient Weight Loss, Delaying The Aging Process, And Enhancing Energy Levels

(A Comprehensive And Systematic Manual For Incorporating A Nutritious Diet Into Your Daily Routine)

Mariusz Ainsworth

TABLE OF CONTENT

The Advantages And Disadvantages Of Fast-Induced Dietary Restriction

For a more comprehensive understanding of the benefits and drawbacks of fasting, it is crucial that you are aware of its effects on the human body. When engaging in a fast, it entails abstaining from the intake of protein, carbohydrates, and minerals, resulting in the absence of these essential nutrients within the body. In a technical context, the initiation of fasting occurs when the human body metabolically switches to utilizing its fat or carbohydrate reserves, as it has depleted all readily available energy from ingested food. It should be noted, however, that in due course, your body will deplete these reserves as well. As the execution of fundamental activities like locomotion and respiration necessitates energy, alternative sources of energy are sought by the body. Subsequently, it shall progress into the protein reservoirs located within the musculature, ultimately infiltrating the vital organs. If such a physiological response occurs in your body, it may lead to a state of malnourishment.

The Pros of Fasting

1) You will experience fat loss and achieve a leaner physique.

The aforementioned phenomenon, wherein your body metabolizes its fat stores during fasting intervals, indicates a beneficial impact. By consistently engaging in intermittent fasting, individuals can expect to experience fat loss and achieve a leaner physique. You will have the ability to attain or move closer to your desired weight and physical appearance.

2) You will have the opportunity to purify your body.

In addition, the human body possesses the capacity to eliminate toxins as it relies on the utilization of fat reserves for energy. In addition to carbohydrates, it is worth noting that the fat depot also comprises chemical compounds that are assimilated from the surrounding environment. These may encompass a synthetic pesticide referred to as DDT which is capable of dispersing within the ecosystem. While engaging in fasting, the human body undergoes the process of burning fat, resulting in the release and subsequent elimination of these chemicals via urine.

3) You will experience an increase in vitality.

Furthermore, you are highly probable to experience an increase in vitality. During the period of fasting, the process of digestion is significantly reduced. Due to the substantial energy demands of the digestive system and the cessation of its functional requirements, it is advisable to allocate your energy towards other physiological processes to optimize utilization. Your body will subsequently utilize the energy to facilitate metabolic processes and support the immune system, thereby contributing to the healing of wounds.

4) There will be a reduction in your Basal Metabolic Rate.

As a consequence of fasting, there will also be a decrease in your BMR or basal metabolic rate. It is of significant importance to acknowledge that the functioning of essential bodily processes like cardiac activity and respiration heavily depends on the basal metabolic rate (BMR). As the basal metabolic rate decreases, typically within a period of one day, there is a concomitant decrease in the core body temperature. Consequently, your body is capable of enhancing its utilization of said energy.

5) Your lifespan will be extended.

Research has demonstrated that caloric restriction is indeed associated with an extension of lifespan. Intermittent fasting operates in a similar fashion to calorie restriction by engaging comparable mechanisms that promote increased lifespan. Consequently, intermittent fasting enhances longevity.

Recent research has revealed that the condition of starvation lends itself to longevity, as the human body adapts in ways that promote enhanced overall well-being. However, it is not necessary to endure prolonged periods of hunger in order to extend one's lifespan. Intermittent fasting enables individuals to savor their preferred culinary delights while experiencing infrequent sensations of hunger. One can acquire the advantages of an extended lifespan without enduring the distress of malnutrition.

6) There will be a decrease in the likelihood of developing cancer.

Although there is a lack of adequate research regarding the correlation between fasting and cancer, preliminary studies present promising results.

An empirical investigation encompassing a sample size of 10 individuals afflicted with cancer has demonstrated that implementing a fasting period prior to the administration of chemotherapy substantially mitigates the adverse effects of the treatment. A separate study corroborated this discovery following the implementation of alternate-day fasting among individuals diagnosed with cancer. It has been determined that abstaining from food before undergoing a treatment leads to improved rates of recovery and reduced mortality.

A multitude of scholarly investigations focused on the relationship between fasting and disease have consistently indicated the advantageous impact of fasting on cardiovascular ailments. Not only does fasting diminish the probabilities of developing cancer, it also mitigates the likelihood of experiencing cardiovascular ailments.

Longer Fasting Regimens

Long fasting regimens are performed with lesser frequency when contrasted with the aforementioned short fasting regimens. This is due to the fact that extended fasting periods exceed 24 hours, consequently lasting for a span of a week or possibly one month, thereby posing challenges in maintaining satiety.

Nevertheless, the decision regarding the most appropriate fasting regimen for an individual ultimately rests with the individual themselves, as there are circumstances in which certain individuals may find prolonged periods of fasting to be more manageable compared to others. Hence, it is recommended that prior to selecting a regimen to pursue, one should experiment with both brief and extended regimens.

If you choose to engage in extended fasting regimens, you will come to realize that by the second day, there will be a noticeable escalation in hunger. Subsequently, hunger levels will progressively escalate over time; however, fortunately, they will eventually diminish as your body undergoes adaptation. It is imperative that you understand the reduction in hunger levels, as this knowledge can serve as a source of motivation to persevere through prolonged periods of fasting without succumbing to temptation. In addition, extended periods of fasting can yield significant advantages, particularly if you have an underlying metabolic issue that requires attention. Below are the prevailing long intermittent fasting regimens:

24-Hour Procedure"

This essentially involves consuming a single meal daily, either from breakfast to breakfast or from dinner to dinner. For instance, if your regular schedule entails having dinner at 8 PM in the evening, then you are limited to consuming one meal solely at 8 PM every day. This does not imply that one must perform this procedure on a daily basis; should it prove challenging, one may opt to implement this intermittent fasting approach on select days throughout the week. In the majority of instances, it is seldom arduous to abstain from consuming food for an entire day, as one typically partakes in sustenance at some point.

It is generally recommended to adhere to this protocol two to three times per week in order to achieve favorable outcomes. If you are able to effectively accomplish this schedule, you may now consider extending the duration to implement this approach.

The Pros

This fasting protocol presents numerous benefits. Firstly, due to its extended duration, this longer fasting protocol exhibits greater efficacy in comparison to shorter fasting protocols.

Furthermore, it aids in economic savings by mitigating the need for expenditures on food. Additionally, you economize on time that would have otherwise been dedicated to meal preparation.

It seamlessly integrates into your daily routine.

It is highly probable that you will experience weight loss, without any significant reduction in lean body mass or muscle, contrary to common concerns.

The cons

This protocol could present challenges for individuals accustomed to consuming meals throughout the day.

Please be advised that in the event you are unable to maintain a continuous duration of 24 hours, but can instead manage a period of 18 to 20 hours, there is no reason for concern. This duration is also deemed acceptable. Continually adapt to the passage of time, and you will successfully endure a 24-hour period without consuming food.

The 5:2 Protocol

According to this protocol, it is required to have regular meals for five days, while for the remaining two days, the allotted caloric intake should not exceed a total of 500 calories. One may consume all of these calories in a singular meal, such as dinner, or alternatively, they can be divided into two portions: breakfast and dinner. This approach exhibits notable resemblances to the 24-hour protocol, albeit with slight variances.

The decision on how to structure your daily schedule rests solely in your hands. One can choose to limit their calorie intake on Monday and Thursday while maintaining a regular diet on the remaining days of the week. Additionally, the option to fast on Tuesday and Thursday, while adhering to a normal eating pattern on the other days, is also available.

Dr. Michael Mosley, a esteemed physician and television producer, gained significant recognition for promoting the technique of intermittent fasting subsequent to his appearance on a renowned BBC program titled "Horizon: Eat, Fast and Live Longer." Although it had sparked intrigue among forward-thinkers such as Brad Pilon and Martin Berkhan, it had not yet captured the attention of the wider audience. Nevertheless, following the release of a BBC documentary and the subsequent publication of the book titled "The Fast Diet," it garnered considerable attention, subsequently leading to the publication of additional books.

The pros

It is relatively effortless for one to incorporate into their daily routine, as the schedule is not excessively demanding.

The cons

It can be challenging to transition back and forth between one's regular dietary routine on a recurring basis.

Intermittent fasting on alternate days

This regimen is alternatively referred to as the eat-stop-eat protocol, wherein one adheres to their regular dietary routine on one day, and then undertakes a fast or significantly restricts calorie intake on the subsequent day. Apart from the fasting pattern, the 5:2 Protocol showcases no significant deviations. Nevertheless, this protocol has undergone extensive research, which is advantageous in terms of ensuring sufficient information. The majority of this research was conducted by Dr. Krista Varady, an assistant professor of nutrition affiliated with the University of Illinois - Chicago. The author penned a publication entitled "The Every Other Day Diet," wherein the majority of her diligent investigation on the subject of alternate day fasting is displayed.

36-Hour Protocol

This fasting regimen involves abstaining from food for a duration of 36 consecutive hours. To illustrate, in the event that you consume dinner at 8 PM on the initial day, it will necessitate abstaining from any further meals on the subsequent day, and solely partaking in breakfast at 8 AM on the third day. Altogether, this would result in a duration of 36 hours of abstaining from food consumption. It is advisable to adhere to this intermittent fasting regimen on two occasions per week.

The pros

It exhibits significantly higher effectiveness compared to shorter fasts, yielding rapid outcomes.

It facilitates rapid weight loss while preserving your lean body mass and muscular integrity.

The cons

It can present a significant challenge to manage, given the necessity of abstaining from food for a duration of 36 hours.

Extended Fasting Periods and Beyond

The 42-hour protocol closely parallels the 36-hour protocol, with a slight extension of 6 hours. For instance, should you choose to have your evening meal at 7 PM on the first day, you would forgo all subsequent meals on the second day and partake in a delayed breakfast or lunch at 12 noon on the third day. You will have successfully abstained from consuming any food or beverages for a continuous duration of 42 hours. In longer fasting regimens, there is no imposition of calorie restrictions during meals, as the decrease in appetite naturally regulates your food intake. This will effectively limit the quantity of calories that you consume. This decline will ensue due to diminished insulin levels, thus there is no reason for concern.

It regulates the functioning of cells, hormones, and genes

The prolonged absence of food results in specific physiological effects on the body. For instance, it will commence the regulation of cellular functioning and induce alterations in hormone levels, thereby facilitating the entry of body fat. Additional alterations that could manifest within the organism comprise:

Insulin levels: there will be a minor decrease in insulin levels, facilitating the body's capacity to metabolize fat.

Elevation of growth hormone in the bloodstream can result in a substantial increase in human growth hormone. Elevated concentrations of this hormone are known to facilitate muscle development and promote fat metabolism.

Cellular Regeneration: The body will initiate the mechanism of cellular repair, encompassing the elimination of cellular waste.

Genetic profiling: Certain advantageous mutations manifest across multiple genes, conferring extended lifespan and bolstering defenses against illnesses.

Reduction in Body Weight and Adipose Tissue

Numerous individuals engage in rapid succession in order to achieve weight loss. In the majority of instances, intermittent fasting will inherently result in a reduced caloric intake. You will ultimately ingest a reduced amount of calories, thereby resulting in the reduction of your body weight. Moreover, fasting enhances the activity of hormones, thus enabling the body to more effectively facilitate weight loss. Decreased levels of growth hormone and insulin facilitate the catabolism of adipose tissue and enhance energy utilization within the body. This is the reason why temporary abstinence from food can lead to a minimum three percent increase in metabolic rate.

From one perspective, it stimulates your metabolic rate to enhance calorie expenditure, simultaneously curbing your food intake. Based on a 2014 review addressing scientific research on intermittent fasting, individuals achieved a weight reduction of approximately 8 percent within a period of fewer than 24 weeks.

It aids in the management of diabetes

Type 2 diabetes has experienced a surge in prevalence in recent years. Any intervention that could mitigate insulin resistance may potentially prove advantageous in decreasing blood glucose levels, thereby affording protection against the development of type 2 diabetes.

Based on several studies conducted on Intermittent Fasting, it has been identified that a notable decrease ranging from three to six percent in blood sugar levels, accompanied by reductions of 21 percent and 31 percent in insulin levels. An investigation conducted on diabetic rats also demonstrated that Intermittent Fasting could play a vital role in safeguarding rats against renal impairment, a prevalent complication faced by individuals with diabetes. This implies that indirect fasting could potentially serve as a viable alternative for individuals with a heightened susceptibility to developing type 2 diabetes.

Simplifying Life

Although this may not be deemed a typical health advantage, it is nevertheless crucial to acknowledge. Numerous individuals opine that adopting temporary fasting can enhance one's quality of life. They are aware that it is necessary to maintain a concerted effort towards nourishment, granted they are granted the liberty to consume sustenance over an extended duration.

They are able to sustain themselves for several days a week without experiencing concerns concerning their nourishment. In general, this dietary regimen has the potential to greatly facilitate your daily routine.

By reducing the workload during the day, enabling oneself to devote attention to other undertakings, one may find themselves inclined to fret over their overall existence. It is widely recognized that stress can adversely affect both our physical well-being and overall quality of life. When one is able to mitigate stress, achieving optimal health becomes effortlessly attainable.

Assistance Available for Cancer

A significant number of individuals are diagnosed with cancer annually. This ailment may give rise to severe circumstances, with its defining features encompassing the unregulated proliferation of cells. Fasting is purported to confer significant advantages related to one's metabolism, thereby potentially diminishing the risk of developing cancer. Several human studies have indicated that fasting has demonstrated potential in mitigating the chemical side effects experienced by cancer patients.

Beneficial for Mental Well-being

Is it possible for an intervention that is effective for the functioning of the human body to also be effective for the functioning of the brain? Fasting has the potential to enhance the metabolic symptoms commonly associated with promoting brain health. This may entail aiding in the management of insulin resistance, the reduction of blood sugar levels, the alleviation of inflammation, and the mitigation of chemical stress.

Numerous investigations have been conducted on rodents, illustrating the potential of intermittent fasting to promote neurogenesis, thereby enhancing cognitive capabilities. Fasting has the potential to enhance and elevate cognitive function. Insufficient presence of this element within the brain can lead to the onset of depression, alongside various other psychological conditions.

It Helps to Improve Cells

The acceleration of our pace can lead to the classification of human cells as the "defensive barrier" during the process of digestion. This process entails the degradation of cells and the catabolism of any proteins that are no longer utilized. As the prevalence of self-medication rises, it can contribute to the prevention of human ailments such as cancer and Alzheimer's disease.

Has the potential to mitigate the onset of Alzheimer's Disease

Alzheimer's is a prevailing neurological condition in contemporary times. The affliction is unremediable, and in order to guarantee your safety from it, the prudence of prevention surpasses remedial measures. According to a particular study which was contacted on rats, one of the ways to prevent the disease is through intermittent fasting.

There are certain instances in which research findings indicate that the incorporation of daily fasting can yield favorable outcomes in the management of Alzheimer's disease. The research has been conducted on both animal subjects and human subjects. In addition to this ailment, scholarly investigations also suggest that intermittent fasting may contribute to the prevention of other ailments such as Parkinson's and Huntington's diseases.

Several case reports indicate that alterations in lifestyle, such as the incorporation of daily or periodic fasting, have shown potential for ameliorating the symptoms associated with Alzheimer's disease in the majority (nine out of ten) of patients. Additionally, research conducted on animals has demonstrated the potential of this fasting regimen to mitigate the onset of other neurodegenerative disorders such as Huntington's disease and Parkinson's disease.

While the majority of these studies were conducted on animals, the outcomes appeared encouraging. Intermittent fasting constitutes a prevailing phenomenon, and the scientific investigation into its underlying mechanisms for promoting wellness is not novel. Acquiring a comprehensive understanding of the advantages of fasting requires a significant amount of time.

Frequent abstaining from food can contribute to an extended lifespan.

One notable aspect of interactive fasting is its potential to contribute to an extended lifespan. Multiple scientific investigations conducted on rodents have demonstrated the potential of intermittent fasting to prolong their lifespan, akin to the effects observed when gradually adhering to a conventional calorie restriction regimen. The observed impact, as illustrated in certain studies, was unexpectedly minimal. An additional factor to consider is that the lifespan of animals that engage in daily fasting is extended by 83% compared to those that do not.

Although there is insufficient empirical evidence from long-term population studies to substantiate the claim that intermittent fasting directly boosts lifespan, it remains a favored concept among individuals seeking to stave off the aging process. Considering the established advantages of the metabolic processes associated with this dietary approach, it is unsurprising that individuals hold the belief that regular fasting can contribute to longevity and overall well-being.

As apparent from the aforementioned, adhering to a fast-food regimen presents numerous advantages. We have only briefly addressed a limited number of them, however, there exists a substantial body of research pertaining to the impact of this dietary regimen and its potential benefits for individuals. Indirect fasting has the potential to enhance various aspects of your life, including one's mental well-being, longevity, weight management, and energy levels.

The 16/8 Method- authored by Martin Berkhan

Ideal for individuals who possess some degree of adaptability in their professional or academic commitments, enabling them to seamlessly anticipate and plan their meals and exercise routine. It is also well-suited for individuals dedicated to their fitness regimen, aiming to reduce body fat while gaining muscle mass.

Commonly referred to as the Lean Gains Protocol, the 16/8 method entails adhering to a restricted feeding window of approximately 8 to 10 hours, with the remaining 14 to 16 hours being designated for fasting on a daily basis. You possess the autonomy to allocate your meals in any manner you see fit within the designated eating period, whether it be two, three, or even multiple meals.

Although a duration of sixteen hours of fasting may appear substantial, it is not. For example, should you choose to consume your final meal of the day at 8pm and subsequently refrain from eating until 12 noon the subsequent day, you will have successfully achieved a 16-hour fasting period. Opting for the 16/8 option would be highly advisable, given that a significant portion of your fasting period will coincide with your sleep schedule. After rousing from slumber, it is permissible to consume coffee, water, or any other non-caloric liquid within the duration of your fasting period.

To optimize this approach, it is advised to incorporate satiating and slowly metabolizing proteins, such as cottage cheese, into your final meal to sustain you during the fasting period.

The pros

The principal advantage of this method lies in its cutting-edge hormonal control, which can be practiced on a daily basis.

Implementing a 16/8 fasting schedule is more advantageous in terms of embracing intermittent fasting as a long-term lifestyle choice due to its regularity and consistent daily adherence.

The 16/8 protocol offers the advantage of facilitating a substantial portion of the fasted state during sleep, thereby enabling the omission of breakfast and minimizing the duration of fasting as a whole.

The Cons

This approach has few disadvantages apart from the fact that it may necessitate a period of adjustment to the practice of omitting breakfast. Please ensure that during meal times, you refrain from exaggerating the portion sizes as this may lead to excessive consumption of food.

Intermittent Fasting on Alternate Days-authored by Dr. James Johnson

Most appropriate for: This protocol is most appropriate for individuals who are following a structured diet plan with a predetermined target weight.

Intermittent fasting, commonly referred to as alternate day fasting or the up day down day diet, entails abstaining from food on alternate days. The preeminent variations for implementing this method involve consuming a total of 500 calories on the designated fasting days, while abstaining entirely from any caloric intake on the remaining fasting days. In essence, one consumes a significantly reduced quantity (approximately one-fifth of the usual amount) to none at all on fasting days, while adhering to a standard diet on non-fasting days. It is recommended that you commence by consuming small amounts on the fasting days and gradually progress towards consuming nothing.

This approach is highly effective for facilitating weight loss; nonetheless, individuals might encounter some challenges when engaging in exercise during the accelerated intervals. You may engage in a gentle physical exercise regime while reserving the rigorous workouts for your usual routine.

The pros

The alternative of observing fasting on alternate days offers considerable flexibility to the majority of individuals, as it allows for effective weekly scheduling.

Engaging in alternate-day fasting entails dedicating half of your week to fasting, thereby considerably enhancing the likelihood of shedding excess weight.

Alternate day fasting similarly adheres to a consistent sequence, facilitating the body's acclimation.

The cons

The imposition of caloric limitations on alternate days could pose greater challenges for certain individuals compared to complete fasting, and there is no assurance that this approach will induce ketosis, a metabolic state characterized by the body relying on ketones as its primary source of energy.

And for individuals who are passionate about fitness, adhering to a calorie deficit on the designated days may present some difficulties.

The 5:2 technique - authored by Michael Mosley

Ideal for: individuals who prioritize their health and face time constraints that hinder adherence to a rigorous meal regimen

This particular form of intermittent fasting entails following a regular diet for a span of five days each week, while limiting calorie consumption to a range of 500 (women) to 600 (men) calories for the remaining two days. You have the option to allocate the calories between lunch and dinner, or distribute them evenly across breakfast, lunch, and dinner, resulting in a reduced portion size for each individual meal. To guarantee optimal performance throughout the week, it is advised to refrain from scheduling consecutive fasting days. You are only required to select two days of the week that are most convenient for you to observe the act of fasting.

While there are no strict guidelines concerning dietary choices, it is essential to bear in mind that consuming food in adherence to a notion of normalcy does not grant unrestricted indulgence in any kind of food. If you desire to achieve success in this endeavor (which I am aware you do), it is imperative that you steer clear of unhealthy foods and instead choose to consume nourishing alternatives.

The pros

This approach necessitates the consumption of 500 to 600 calories during the designated 'fast' days, thereby affording you greater ease.

It is particularly beneficial for novice individuals as it allows for consumption of a modest meal (within the range of 500 to 600 calories) on days designated for fasting.

The cons

The dietary regimen lacks coherence in that it fails to specify the fasting days, thus rendering it more challenging to adhere to and maintain the prescribed method.

Furthermore, there is a likelihood of surpassing the recommended daily calorie intake during the 48-hour period of 'fasting', particularly when opting for nutritionally unfavorable food choices that are inherently calorie-dense.

Intermittent Fasting Protocols

The Eat-Stop-Eat Method

This method requires abstaining from the intake of any edibles or liquids for a period of 24 hours. You are granted the opportunity to partake in this endeavor either once or twice per week. In this particular method, an individual can partake in a meal within a specific timeframe, after which they refrain from eating until the corresponding hour on the subsequent day, thus effectively accomplishing a full 24-hour fasting period. An example of this concept involves partaking in a customary midday meal at 1pm, followed by an abstention from eating until the following day at 1pm, at which point one reinitiates their regular dietary practices.

It is imperative to recognize that this approach can pose a significant difficulty for individuals who possess limited experience. To mitigate the feeling of hunger, one may choose to ingest water or other calorie-free beverages while abstaining from eating. As a beginner, it is acceptable for you to exercise discernment in strictly adhering to a 24-hour schedule. Adopting an initial timeframe of either 12 or 14 hours, and subsequently extending it progressively, would be deemed as an appropriate strategy until you can effectively conform to the intended timetable.

The most efficient approach to address this issue would involve partaking in your meals during the early hours of the day, for instance at 8am, and then observing a period of abstinence from food until 8am the next day. This approach is advisable as it will mitigate your hunger sensations throughout the day. Furthermore, during your state of slumber, the inevitable sensation of hunger is likely to manifest.

The Leangains Protocol

This is commonly known as the 16/8 method due to its utilization of a 16-hour fasting period coupled with an 8-hour window for meal consumption on a daily basis. It was formulated and disseminated by a Swedish nutritionist named Martin Berkhan. In accordance with the principles of the leangains methodology, individuals begin their dietary regimen by partaking in a meal at a prescribed hour, followed by another sustenance prior to the culmination of an eight-hour timeframe. Subsequently, you refrain from consuming food for the consecutive 16 hours, thus encompassing a cumulative duration of 24 hours for the combined periods of eating and fasting. As an example, one could choose to abstain from breakfast and opt for lunch at 12.30pm, followed by supper at 8.30pm, in order to uphold a consistent 8-hour gap between meals. Following that, it is feasible to refrain from consuming any food for the subsequent 16-hour duration until the subsequent lunchtime at 12.30pm.

Leangains is predominantly employed by athletes and individuals seeking to attain a finely sculpted physique through athletic training. Furthermore, the protocol includes guidelines pertaining to appropriate dietary selections for both days dedicated to physical exertion and days of rest. In particular, for individuals engaging in physical exercise, the advisable practice is to incorporate protein-rich foods, such as meat, into their diet alongside a variety of vegetables and fruits for the purpose of breaking the fast. For optimal preparation for physical exercise, it is recommended to incorporate carbohydrates, such as starches like whole wheat bread or potatoes. It is advisable to partake in a substantial period of physical exercise after finishing this meal, followed by a subsequent meal consisting of complex carbohydrates, potentially accompanied by a preferred dessert, such as ice cream. It is recommended, though, to choose low-fat options. Within the period of your designated rest, you may reduce your calorie intake by effectively reducing your consumption of carbohydrates, preferring instead to prioritize vegetables and meat as the primary constituents of your dietary plan.

This methodology is widely pervasive and holds the capability to generate substantial outcomes in the enhancement of your muscle.

The Rapid Dietary Approach

It is also commonly known as the 5:2 diet. This methodology advocates for adhering to a consistent dietary regimen for a duration of five days, subsequently implementing a regime of restricting calorie consumption to a range of 500-600 calories for two days on a weekly basis. Kindly ensure that there is no consecutive arrangement of days. It is recommended that males consume 600 calories, while females are encouraged to consume 500 calories during the fasting period.

Hence, this protocol does not entail a total prohibition on meal consumption, but rather substantially curtails the quantity during your fasting days.

For instance, it is possible to adhere to a consistent eating regimen throughout the week, except on Wednesdays and Fridays. On these fasting days, two small meals can be consumed, each amounting to only half of the total calories needed during the fasting period. Consequently, it follows that males should consume 300 calories, while females should consume 250 calories on every fasting day.

Approach towards Voluntary Refraining from Food Consumption

This method can be regarded as an impromptu and unstructured procedure, in which there is no obligatory requirement to strictly adhere to a predetermined eating or fasting timetable. Within this particular framework, there exists no requirement to strictly follow a designated fasting routine. You partake in fasting only when you are fully satisfied and devoid of any sensation of hunger. From time to time, a scenario may occur wherein an individual experiences a sense of fullness and consequently chooses to abstain from their midday meal until the subsequent evening dining occasion. In the days to come, you might not feel inclined to partake in breakfast due to time constraints, leading to its omission. When partaking in this activity, you are essentially adopting a method of unstructured or sporadic periodic fasting.

The Methodological Approach of the Warrior Diet

As suggested by its designation, this involves consuming sustenance comparable to that of a respected warrior or soldier. This method involves the consumption of moderate servings of fresh fruits and vegetables throughout the day, followed by a substantial meal in the evening.

The warrior diet, in essence, involves refraining from consuming your customary substantial meals such as breakfast and lunch. Conversely, you constrain your consumption to a limited assortment of fruits and vegetables, which furnish nourishment until your habitual evening meal. Fruits and vegetables are extensively acknowledged for their nutritional advantages and reduced caloric value. This particular approach may serve as an optimum solution for individuals adhering to the intermittent fasting regimen.

What potential benefits can be obtained by adhering to an intermittent fasting regimen? Now, let us progress to the examination and analysis of the aforementioned elements.

The Efficacy Of Intermittent Fasting In Promoting Healthier Skin

The secret to achieving skin that is radiant, youthful, and resilient does not lie in external factors. While it is possible to invest in costly beauty products in order to enhance the appearance of your skin, it is important to note that they cannot fully repair its overall health. For individuals seeking to attain radiant and healthy skin, it is imperative to delve deeper into one's internal well-being. The food one consumes largely determines the manner in which their body experiences sensations and operates. The majority of cosmetic products often contain chemicals, and their application to our facial skin can be likened to utilizing a Band-Aid to address a profound injury.

Were you aware that the human body houses the largest organ known as the skin? It encompasses an estimated area of approximately 2 square meters, constituting approximately 20% of the overall body mass in an adult human. The integumentary system serves as a barrier, shielding the internal human system from the external environment. The human skin consists of two distinct layers, namely the epidermis and the dermis. The uppermost layer of skin is known as the epidermis, while the lower layer is referred to as the dermis. These two layers of skin are distinctly segregated by a basement membrane. The dermis is additionally segmented into five subsidiary layers. In addition to the dermis and epidermis, there exists another significant stratum referred to as the hypodermis. The hypodermis comprises adipose tissue and various other types of connective tissues.

In totality, the integumentary system comprises approximately seven layers, however, our attention is primarily focused on the superficial layer that is perceptible to sight. It should be clarified that abstaining from purchasing skin products altogether is not advised; however, those genuinely seeking to enhance their skin's appearance are encouraged to introspect. It is highly advisable to devise a lasting solution in order to enhance the overall health of your skin, rather than opting for temporary remedies.

The hypodermis can be understood as a stratum comprised mainly of connective tissue and elastin. The hypodermis primarily functions as a dampener for impacts, a heat insulator for the body, and a storage site for energy. The regions characterized by the greatest thickness of the hypodermis involve the buttocks, soles of the feet, and palms of the hands. As one advances in age, the hypodermis undergoes atrophy, leading to the manifestation of wrinkles. Therefore, aging can be defined as the gradual accumulation of tissue damage over time. Glycation is the main cause of such damage.

Prior to familiarizing yourself with the ways in which fasting can enhance the health of your skin, it is imperative to acquire a comprehensive understanding of several key terms, which are enumerated as follows.

Collagen

The integumentary system consists of a protein called collagen, which functions to provide structural support and cohesion to the skin. Collagen represents the protein that is most prevalent within the human body. Were you aware that approximately 75% of the overall composition of the skin consists of collagen?

Elastin

An additional significant protein present in the skin, along with connective tissue, is elastin. Elastin plays a predominant role in facilitating the resilient action of the skin. Elastic skin consistently reverts to its initial form when gently compressed or tugged upon. Insufficient presence of elastin may result in skin laxity. Elastin facilitates the maintenance of skin smoothness, even when subjected to stretching. It facilitates the performance of typical activities such as engaging in muscle contractions during exercise.

Glucose

Glucose serves as the principal energy source for the human body. The human body metabolizes sugar, carbohydrates, and sometimes an excess of protein into glucose. Nevertheless, in cases where the body fails to adequately metabolize glucose, it gives rise to various deleterious repercussions. The glucose molecules have the ability to initiate the process of forming bonds with unbound protein molecules such as elastin and collagen. This phenomenon is characterized by a gradual and progressive impairment of the tissue's elasticity within the body, and it is commonly referred to as glycation.

Glycation

Glycation refers to the enzymatic process by which a saccharide molecule initiates a chemical union with either a lipid or a polypeptide molecule. Glycation is additionally regarded as a biological indicator for various health conditions such as diabetes and aging.

What are the effects of the aging process?

With the passage of time, the dermal layer undergoes a thinning process. This phenomenon commonly occurs in females and is particularly noticeable on regions such as the upper thorax, facial area, cervical region, hands, and anterior portions of the lower arms. As one ages, there is a diminishment in the body's capacity to generate collagen. The efficacy of fibroblast cells responsible for collagen production declines. In females, there is a gradual decline in estrogen production following menopause, which subsequently accelerates the progression of skin aging. In addition, there is a decrease in keratin-producing cells. Keratin constitutes a vital architectural constituent of the integumentary system, and the deterioration of this constituent results in a diminishment of the skin's inherent luminosity.

Therefore, what is the negative impact of sugar on one's health?

The overabundance of sugar or sugar molecules that are not efficiently metabolized result in glycation. AGEs, known as Advanced Glycation End Products, are formed as a result of the process of glycation. Nearly everything within the human body comprises a certain type of protein or another. Glycation adversely impacts all varieties of proteins. Hair, skin, nails, flesh, organs, muscles, and every other constituent element you may conceive are all comprised of protein.

When proteins, such as elastin and collagen, undergo glycation, they exhibit diminished elasticity, rigidity, and impaired regenerative capacity. Consequent to these factors, the skin experiences cracking, thinning, and loosening. As a result of glycation, the oxidation of other proteins occurs, leading to the loss of their regenerative properties. Inflammation is responsible for inducing oxidative damage. Inflammation can severely compromise the overall health of your skin. Chronic inflammation negatively impacts the structural elements of the skin, such as elastin and collagen, leading to damage. These factors culminate in the development of wrinkles, skin laxity, and the emergence of fine lines. Furthermore, it is noteworthy that the immunological reaction within your body could potentially instigate various dermatological ailments such as acne, rosacea, and even urticaria.

Autophagy plays a crucial role in enhancing the regeneration of impaired skin, and one of the most effective approaches to initiate autophagy is through the practice of intermittent fasting. Autophagy serves as the fundamental physiological process by which the body eliminates various toxins present internally, alongside the restoration of cellular damage. Additionally, it retards the aging process and preserves cellular youth and vitality. Autophagy exerts an impact on diverse facets of one's well-being, encompassing the process of aging, the vitality of the dermis, and body mass composition. As a result of a multitude of factors, the process of autophagy progressively decelerates. When the process of autophagy begins to decelerate, the capacity of the body to effectively detoxify and rejuvenate itself diminishes. All of this renders you increasingly vulnerable to the deleterious effects of the aging process. The integrity of your skin may be compromised as a result of factors such as stress, dietary habits, sun exposure, and the presence of harmful substances. When autophagy operates at its peak efficiency, the body is able to initiate the mending of the skin and subsequently substitute any afflicted cells. Nevertheless, in the absence of autophagy activation, the capacity to mitigate skin aging-related damage is rendered futile. Additionally, it leads to heightened inflammation and diminishes the body's capacity to generate collagen and other crucial structural constituents as elaborated in the preceding segment.

The process of skin aging and damage occurs as a result of the accumulation of impaired proteins within the body, coupled with an inability to effectively eliminate these damaged cells. By eliciting autophagy, it aids in cellular clearance and diminishes skin damage.

Fasting aids in the release of various toxins that are present within the body and initiates an internal cleansing of the colon. Through this action, your body can efficiently assimilate a greater amount of nutrients from the sustenance you ingest. Hence, it is imperative that you consume nutritious and well-balanced meals whenever you conclude your period of abstinence. When your physical well-being is optimized and devoid of harmful substances, it contributes to the enhancement of your skin's aesthetic qualities. Fasting additionally purges toxins from your body. Toxins are the primary factor responsible for the occurrence of hormonal imbalances, in conjunction with the provocation of irritation. These two factors are the predominant catalysts for the occurrence of skin breakouts. Fasting has been noted to effectively mitigate acne breakouts and augment the body's capacity to heal acne scars. Intermittent fasting exhibits efficacy in managing blood sugar levels and enhancing the functionality of the gut microbiota. These factors play an indirect role in the amelioration of inflammatory skin conditions such as eczema and acne.

Commence practicing mindful eating habits to uphold a harmonious appearance of your skin. One can adopt a dietary approach that involves the consumption of antioxidant-rich foods, coupled with the reduction of inflammatory food intake, as a straightforward means to address this issue. The different ingredients you must avoid are sugar, saturated fats, trans fats, Omega-6 fatty acids, refined carbs, gluten, casein, and MSG. The various food items abundant in antioxidants comprise of dark chocolate, blueberries, strawberries, goji berries, raspberries (or any other type of berries), artichokes, pecans, kale, spinach, and beetroot. Additional sources of antioxidants comprise green tea, sweet potatoes, dark green leafy vegetables, whole grains, fish, and various legumes in the diet. Through the augmentation of your consumption of food items abundant in antioxidants, you can effectively neutralize the detrimental effects induced by inflammatory food sources.

The Warrior Diet

As you might have discerned from the nomenclature of the protocol, it aims to replicate the dietary practices of esteemed warriors from antiquity. Specifically, it embraces the notion that the warriors of ancient times did not consume multiple small meals interspersed throughout the day. Instead, they partook in two substantial meals per day limited to a maximum. The individual behind the protocol, Ori Hofmekler, advises practicing daily fasting for a period of up to 20 hours, with the consumption of food limited to a four-hour timeframe solely during the evening.

There is a certain concern that many dedicated fasters have with this particular protocol, which pertains to the concept of fasting itself. You see, within the framework of this protocol, fasting does not pertain to complete abstinence from food but rather pertains to caloric restriction, specifically consuming minimal quantities of food. Therefore, it is possible to consume minor quantities of specific foods during the 20-hour fasting period on a daily basis without experiencing extreme hunger.

Strategies for Enacting the Warrior Diet

To be frank, there is limited practical application taking place in this context except for:

Consume modest portions of lean proteins, vegetables, or fruits throughout the day while fasting; and

Indulge in a satisfying meal during a limited four-hour period in the evening, prior to retiring for the night.

It is important to recognize that fruit juice that is readily available for purchase does not qualify as a serving of fruit. When consuming fruit juice, it is advisable to opt for freshly squeezed variations rather than those that are laden with excessive amounts of sugar.

Nevertheless, there exist certain regulations to adhere to regarding the types of food that are permissible for consumption. This phenomenon can be attributed to the prevailing notion that the human body necessitates specific nutrients to facilitate an optimal state of rest and recuperation during the period of sleep. In addition, it necessitates the consumption of meals during nighttime, as it purportedly enhances the body's parasympathetic nervous system functionality, facilitating rest, rejuvenation, recovery, and thorough digestion of food. Consequently, these factors contribute to enhancing the body's capacity to generate human growth hormones, which play a vital role in facilitating fat reduction and preserving or developing muscular tissue.

An additional stipulation pertaining to this protocol is the prescribed sequence of meals during nighttime. Hofmekler advises prioritizing the consumption of vegetables initially, followed by the intake of dietary fat and protein. Should you experience lingering hunger, you have the option to satiate it by consuming additional portions of fruit during the remaining four-hour timeframe.

Benefits of the Warrior Diet

A key benefit of the Warrior Diet, which has faced criticism from dedicated fasters, lies in its avoidance of strict fasting, instead focusing on controlled consumption of specific food groups. This greatly enhances the tolerability factor for a significant number of individuals, even amidst a daily period of under-eating lasting 20 hours. Beneath the Warrior Diet, you will be alleviated from the concern of enduring sensations of hunger.

Another benefit of the Warrior Diet lies in its inherent simplicity. One should simply consume small portions of raw vegetables, fruits, and lean protein intermittently during the day while indulging in one to two substantial meals during the evening. That's it. The more straightforward something is, the more manageable it becomes to maintain.

Drawbacks of the Warrior Diet

The drawbacks of the Warrior Diet could be deemed as insubstantial. One of these factors pertains to the relatively minor inconvenience of having to adhere to a specific dietary regimen during your evening meals and periods of under consumption, wherein certain types of food must be consumed in a designated order or sequence. However, it can be argued that it is a regrettable justification for a so-called "disadvantage."

Another drawback is that it may interfere with your social interactions. Why? This is primarily due to the fact that the majority of social gatherings or get-togethers entail the inclusion of food or beverages, such as meals, refreshments, dining experiences, or coffee engagements. With that being stated, it is possible that your availability is limited to a four-hour period during the evening designated for meals. Unless you can guarantee the ability to consume limited portions of vegetables, fruits, or lean protein during your daytime engagements.

A significant drawback, particularly during the initial stages, revolves around the necessity of obtaining the majority, if not all, of your daily caloric requirements within one or two substantial meals in the evening. This can present a particular challenge in the case where one is accustomed to consuming frequent small meals daily or engaging in the habit of consuming substantial and regular snacks throughout the day.

Fortunately, there is the option of gradually acclimating oneself to the protocol over a span of several weeks or months. Commence by gradually elevating the caloric intake for your evening meal, while concurrently reducing the proportion of food consumed during breakfast and lunch. Gradual modifications over a prolonged duration have the potential to enable eventual acclimatization.

If it becomes apparent that consuming an adequate amount of calories through two substantial meals poses a challenge due to the considerable volume of food required, you may consider augmenting your meals with high-calorie alternatives such as virgin coconut oil or medium chain triglycerides (MCT) oil. Both of these products boast a significant caloric content, to the extent that incorporating one or two tablespoons into your evening consumption can effectively provide the necessary supplementary calories required to sustain optimal energy levels throughout your day. An advantageous characteristic of these oils lies in their negligible impact on insulin sensitivity and blood sugar levels, thereby facilitating sustained energy levels without subsequent depletion.

Appropriate Actions To Undertake While Fasting

During the fasting period, it is probable that you will still be ingesting a specific quantity. With the exception of dry fasting, which entails consuming nothing, this is generally confined to beverages with zero calorie content. For specific fasting practices, or among particular individuals who choose to fast, a prescribed caloric intake may also be permissible (typically in the range of 500-600 calories per day). Regardless of the specific type of fast you adhere to, it is important to exercise caution in your dietary habits during the period when you resume eating, after having invested considerable effort in your fasting routine. For the purpose of gaining a more thorough comprehension of the acceptable and unacceptable practices associated with consuming food whilst adhering to a fasting regimen, the ensuing portion will highlight certain particulars.

What to consume

When the sensation of hunger arises, or when there is a desire to consume nourishment while observing a fast, viable alternatives are available. Perhaps you are spending time in the company of acquaintances or relatives who are indulging in food, and partaking in something suitable for your consumption could be beneficial. Alternatively, it is possible that treating yourself to a small and pleasurable delicacy is what you require. Below are several alternatives that are suitable for inclusion in your diet plan.

Unadulterated black coffee, without any sweetener or cream. Coffee occupies the foremost position among fasting consumables due to its inherent merits. Caffeinated beverages enhance the process of autophagy and suppress appetite. It not only fails to impede fasting, but rather, it can facilitate the effectiveness of your fast. Do not hesitate to indulge in a cup of coffee in the morning or evening! However, exercise caution by refraining from the addition of sweeteners, including artificial ones. Similar to sugar, artificial sweeteners elicit a response in the body that triggers an increase in insulin levels, potentially disrupting the fasting state.

Any variant of tea, be it green tea, herbal tea, or black tea, is equally gratifying. The solitary consideration entails refraining from adding any substances with caloric content and abstaining from incorporating artificial sweeteners, much like what is advised for coffee.

Diet sodas- It is advisable to refrain from consuming any type of soda, including diet sodas. However, if you feel compelled to indulge, opting for diet soda is a more suitable choice. In a manner analogous to coffee, the consumption of sweeteners can elicit a surge in insulin levels. When making a selection of a diet soda, please consider opting for a product that employs Stevia as a sweetening agent. Due to its natural composition, Stevia is less prone to trigger a sudden surge in insulin levels. Zevia brand sodas provide an excellent alternative that is devoid of calories and artificial sweeteners.

Water is universally permissible, unless one is undertaking a dry fast. Maintaining proper hydration is a beneficial practice and there is no justification for deviating from it during the fasting period. Indeed, the consumption of water can serve to mitigate the adverse consequences of hunger and satiate the innate impulse to ingest sustenance.

Nutrition - If you are adhering to a fast that permits limited caloric consumption, it is advisable to prioritize food choices that are rich in fiber and protein. These options can promote satiety while minimizing excessive caloric intake. Soup presents itself as an excellent choice in this regard, as its high liquid content contributes to satiety while consuming fewer quantities of food.

What not to consume

The substances you abstain from consuming are of equal importance to the ones you choose to ingest while observing a period of fasting. After reviewing the provisions for consumption during fasting intervals, presented herewith is a concise manual outlining particular items that it may be advisable to abstain from.

Food

In general, this should be quite evident. When engaged in a fast, it is evident that consuming food is clearly prohibited. During non-fasting periods, it is advisable to refrain from incorporating additional unhealthy foods. Do not allow your mind to persuade you that fasting provides justification for indulging in unhealthy eating habits subsequently. Consuming a regular diet involves consuming the same range of food that would have been eaten had a period of fasting not been undertaken.

Branch Amino Acids (BCAAs)

Furthermore, it is essential to be mindful of Branch Chain Amino Acids during a period of fasting. These supplements have been proven effective in promoting muscle growth, which has generated some contention regarding the combination of BCAAs and fasting. In fasting periods, it is imperative to refrain from consuming BCAA's as they have the potential to disrupt the fasting state. Branched-chain amino acids (BCAAs) possess caloric content and elicit insulin secretion. However, this does not imply that you are prohibited from consuming them during your fasting period. Simply exercise mindfulness with respect to them.

BCAAs do not elicit an influx of insulin, and owing to their ability to preserve muscle mass, it might be advisable for you to persist in their consumption during your fasting phase. Similar to the decision between fasting with a calorie intake of 500-600 per day or completely abstaining from food, this is a matter of personal preference in terms of how one wishes to approach their fasting practice. Should you choose not to consume them during your fasting period, it remains permissible to intake them during your consumption periods. Consequently, it is unnecessary to halt the usage of these supplements in either case.

When to work out

If you have chosen to adopt intermittent fasting, it is likely that you are aiming to enhance your physical condition. For many individuals, this entails the development of muscle mass to the same extent as the reduction of body weight. Regardless of whether your goal is not to enhance muscle mass, it remains essential to uphold strength and well-being, which necessitates engaging in physical activity.

Engaging in physical activity of any form is beneficial for one's health. If you are able to arrive promptly, then any instance of doing so will prove advantageous for you. Nevertheless, if your goal is to optimize your influence, engaging in training sessions while in a state of fasting is the preferred approach.

When engaging in physical exercise while fasting, it is crucial to be cognizant of the timing of the fast as it can have an impact. At the culmination of your fasting period, you will experience the highest rate of caloric expenditure; however, concurrently, you will also encounter pronounced fatigue, thereby impeding the ease and intensity of your workouts, making them considerably more strenuous and draining. Exercising earlier during the fasting period allows you to retain residual energy from previous meals. For numerous individuals, this leads to a more pleasurable exercise session and justifies the trade-off of experiencing a slightly heightened level of exertion. The decision regarding what is more effective for your physical well-being and mental state rests in your hands.

In the event that exercising during a fasting period yields unsatisfactory results or if an individual possesses the necessary time and energy to engage in both activities, certain principles can be applied to maximize the efficacy of workouts conducted post-fast. Engaging in physical exercise immediately after a meal may not be the optimal decision. Following a period of fasting, the circulation of blood in your body will facilitate the process of digestion.

Consuming food immediately results in the diversion of the blood supply. Consequently, if you engage in physical exercise too soon after a meal, it will result in reduced absorption of nutrients from your food. Please refrain from immediately engaging in physical activity until you have allowed yourself sufficient time to process and assimilate the information.

Maximizing Efficiency and Enjoyment in your IF Endeavors with Effective Strategies

The limited number of individuals who can consistently engage in fasting over an extended period stems from their inability to grasp the concept of deriving enjoyment from it. Presented herewith are strategies that can be employed to ensure that your fasting endeavors are enjoyable while yielding the desired outcomes:

Strategy #1: Disregard the notion of specific working hours; instead, prioritize the duration of time intervals, without attaching undue importance to them.

The majority of individuals tend to rise early in order to attend to their work obligations, consequently experiencing challenges in observing the fast due to the early hours of awakening. They will arise at either 5am or 6am and endeavor to abstain from consuming any food until 1pm, as they have been instructed to partake of their initial meal at approximately that hour.

Indeed, the dynamics of the game vary contingent upon the time at which one awakens in the morning. If you arise at the hour of 11 am, it logically ensues that you must continue your fast until after 1pm, unless you consumed your evening meal ahead of schedule the night prior. Similarly, if one arises at 5am, it is unnecessary to delay one's lunch until 1pm. If one adheres to a 16/8 regimen and arises at 5am, it would be acceptable to consume meals between the hours of 10am to 12pm.

It should be noted that the human body does not inherently distinguish specific 8-hour feeding windows or 16-hour fasting periods; therefore, abstaining from food intake for a duration of 7 hours and 33 minutes will not yield detrimental effects. Moreover, prolonging the duration of your fast beyond 8 hours will have no adverse consequences.

While it is important to approach the hours with due diligence, it is equally crucial to uphold an appropriate level of seriousness in order to maintain the recommended fasting duration.

Alternate Approach #2: Employ caffeine as a strategic asset.

Indeed, water proves to be an ally during periods of fasting. However, in reality, caffeine can prove to be an even more valuable ally. Many adherents of fasting assert that the consumption of caffeine facilitated their affinity for the practice. Caffeine exhibits significantly greater potency when consumed while in a state of fasting. Furthermore, caffeine amplifies several of the impacts of fasting. Caffeine generally has a profound effect on one's metabolism, suppressing the appetite and significantly enhancing energy levels. Additionally, caffeine enhances the process of fat mobilization and enhances cognitive clarity and acuity.

With that being stated, it is crucial to employ caffeine in a strategic manner—relying on a coffee mug as a constant companion during the fasting period will ultimately prove counterproductive. Should you develop a habit of consuming substantial quantities of coffee or tea throughout the day, it is inevitable that your body will gradually build a tolerance to the stimulant effects of caffeine. As time elapses, the capacity of the appetite-suppressing impact will diminish alongside the energy-enhancing effect.

Hence, it is advised to decrease your consumption of caffeine to its minimum level, and furthermore, it is recommended to abstain from the practice of consuming coffee in large quantities in order to avoid the body's development of tolerance towards caffeine.

Allow me to offer a suggestion: consume two modestly-sized black coffee mugs within your designated fasting period, refraining from coffee consumption for the remaining duration. If you happen to desire a hot beverage at a later point in the day, herbal tea can be considered a favorable choice.

Strategy number three: Engage in strategic physical activity.

This is essential literature for individuals who have a proclivity towards vigorous exercise. Autonomous of other factors, intermittent fasting demonstrates remarkable efficacy in promoting fat loss. Furthermore, it is worth noting that your energy levels during the initial weeks of fasting may be comparatively lower compared to both your usual state and the days when you are not fasting. Sure enough, this will soon get rectified, but what is the point of combining fasting with intense exercise, to the point where your body begins attacking and burning lean muscle to provide sufficient energy for the taxing internal environment you are creating?

Intermittent fasting exercises should be structured around low-volume resistance training for the purpose of developing strength and muscle mass, and low-intensity cardiovascular activities like leisurely walks can be employed solely to facilitate calorie burning and weight reduction. If you are determined to engage in conditioning exercises, it is advisable to limit your activities to brief sprints lasting no longer than 30 minutes.

Unless one possesses the attributes of a competitive athlete, there is no need to undertake any additional measures beyond this. If you desire to engage in additional physical activity, it is important to ensure that it is maintained at a moderate to low intensity level.

Strategic Approach #4: Consume fruits judiciously as snacks

There will be frequent instances when you may experience hunger, with a considerable amount of time remaining until your initial meal can be consumed. When encountering such circumstances, it is advisable to indulge in the consumption of a piece of fruit. Fruits are highly advantageous during periods of fasting as they effectively replenish liver glycogen stores. Signals are transmitted to the brain, inducing hunger, when there is an extended period of depletion in liver glycogen levels caused by a lack of food.

By consuming a portion of fruit towards the conclusion of your fasting period, you are effectively suppressing your appetite cues, thereby facilitating the successful completion of your fasting regimen on a consistent basis. Through the passage of time, you will encounter amplified outcomes through this process. And furthermore, the restoration of liver glycogen will effectively transition your body back into a state of anabolism.

The optimal time to consume fruit is when one's stomach is relatively void of food and carbohydrate reserves are depleted. This guarantees that instead of being stored as adipose tissue, the carbohydrates obtained from the fruit are promptly utilized to restore hepatic glycogen.

Physical Fitness Regimen And Monitoring Advancements

Are you aware that engaging in physical activity without having consumed any food is advantageous for the body, as it promotes both physical fitness and overall well-being? During a period of fasting, the metabolic functioning of the human body can experience enhancements of up to fivefold. When undergoing training in a state of fasting, the enhanced metabolic processes within your body stimulate the accelerated degradation of fat and glycogen, thereby supplying the body with essential energy. As a consequence, it is feasible to efficiently engage in physical activity even during a period of fasting.

In the following chapter, we will address a range of significant considerations and queries that may arise pertaining to exercise and intermittent fasting. Next, we shall proceed to present methods for monitoring and evaluating your progress while engaging in fasting.

Exercise and IF

What is the appropriate way to engage in physical activity while observing a period of fasting?

Primarily, gaining a comprehensive understanding of your intermittent fasting strategy is crucial prior to embarking on a workout regimen. As an illustration, one may experience considerable fatigue nearing the conclusion of the fasting period in a 5:2

dietary regimen, yet observe a notable surge in energy levels while adhering to the Leangains approach.

Safety is of paramount significance.

It is advisable to ensure that you are in a satisfactory physical condition before initiating exercise in a state of fasting. If you are experiencing a level of physical weakness that hinders your ability to be highly productive, it is advisable to forgo that exercise session. Nevertheless, it should be noted that one can still engage in physical activity even in the absence of consuming a meal beforehand. When executed correctly, exercise regimens serve as the perfect supplementary component to any intermittent fasting methodology.

The meals factor

Dr. Vincent Padre of Padre Integrative Health stresses the importance of planning your meals around your workouts. Padre advises that it is preferable to engage in cardiovascular exercises in a fasted state. Cardiovascular exercises encompass any form of physical activity that elevates the heart rate. It is imperative to incorporate a dinner into your meal planning that will sufficiently fuel your body for the physical demands of the subsequent day's exercise regimen. This approach serves as a means to enhance your state of readiness.

Which exercises would be recommended for you to engage in?

At this location, you have the opportunity to engage in aerobic exercises, strength training, and gentle stretching.

Aerobic exercises can be defined as cardiovascular exercises aimed at providing a stimulus to the heart and lungs, consequently heightening one's endurance capabilities. Aerobic exercises additionally assist in the relaxation of blood vessel walls, the reduction of harmful LDL cholesterol levels, the mitigation of inflammation, and the promotion of body fat burning. Additional instances of aerobic exercises comprise of fast-paced walking, swimming, running, and engaging in dance movements. Over time, these exercises enhance the risk factors linked to heart disease and help regulate insulin levels. Additionally, they provide insulation against various other chronic ailments such as breast cancer, colorectal cancer, and depressive disorders. Make an effort to uphold a goal of engaging in 150 minutes of exercise on a weekly basis.

Strength training aids in the process of muscular restoration, facilitating the body's ability to regain previously lost muscle mass. Engaging in strength training will not solely augment your efficiency in performing everyday activities, but also foster bone development, reduce blood sugar levels, and facilitate the burning of surplus fat, contributing to weight reduction. Enhancing muscular tonicity additionally enhances your equilibrium and body alignment. Strength training exercises encompass activities such as squats, pushups, lunges, and a range of resistance exercises. You have the option to consult a physiotherapist to develop a personalized fitness regimen for your needs. The physiotherapist will guide you through a range of tips and techniques aimed at optimizing the execution of these exercises.

Engaging in stretching exercises is beneficial for the preservation of your body's flexibility. This is the point at which the influence of age becomes significant. As individuals grow older, there is a natural tendency for muscles and tendons to undergo a shortening process. This, in turn, contributes to a decline in flexibility and increases vulnerability to potential risks and hazards. Potential risks encompass muscular cramping, joint discomfort, and bodily rigidity. These conditions give rise to difficulties in performing basic movements such as bending and maintaining an upright sitting posture, requiring substantial effort. A program that facilitates stretching on alternate days or a minimum of four times per week is considered beneficial to engage in.

Tracking Your Progress

The objective of monitoring your progress is to ensure that you are making steady progress toward your stated objectives. Given that you are already undertaking the arduous task, it is advisable to refrain from unnecessarily complicating the process of documenting your journal entries. While there exist numerous methods for tracking those figures, we shall now present the prevailing approaches:

Take your measurements

Affordability is not a constraint in this matter. A tape measure of affordable price available at a local retail establishment will suffice. It is advisable to obtain your measurements prior to commencing a workout regimen, ideally in the morning or during the optimal timeframe determined by the specific fasting protocol you have embraced. No matter what you are measuring, whether it be the circumference of your biceps, neck, hips, chest, or shoulders, it is imperative that you maintain honesty in recording your measurements. Strive to diligently record the precise observations portrayed on the scale, avoiding any personal bias towards the desired measurement outcome.

Calculate the ratio of adipose tissue in relation to total body mass.

This can pose a challenge for individuals seeking precise numerical data. Nonetheless, if financial constraints are a concern, employing a basic body fat caliper would prove sufficient. If you do not have any reservations about allocating a monthly budget, you may consider enrolling in a fitness facility where you can have your body metrics evaluated. In my opinion, the more economical alternative is still effective in accomplishing the task.

Track your calories

We cannot overemphasize this. The success of weight loss and muscle building endeavors is contingent upon the quantity of calories one ingests. Having expressed that, there exist methods to assist in controlling your calorie intake. Having a clear understanding of one's dietary preferences, and acknowledging that individuals often have repetitive eating patterns, facilitates the meticulous monitoring of every calorie ingested. If you have a preference for manual tracking, there is no issue with recording it in a journal. There exist digital alternatives, encompassing applications and websites specifically designed for this purpose, such as www.dailyplate.com and the My Fitness app.

The Advantages Of Practicing Intermittent Fasting

Intermittent fasting has the potential to enhance mental clarity and increase physical strength...

Ezra Taft Benson

I have elucidated the reasons for prioritizing intermittent fasting over alternative dietary regimens. Now, may I provide you with a comprehensive overview of the precise health advantages associated with the practice of intermittent fasting?

Effective weight loss

Obesity stands as a paramount health concern in the early years of the twenty-first century. According to data from the CDC, more than 45 million individuals in the United States undertake dietary measures each year with the aim of shedding weight. Surprisingly, a staggering 70% of Americans over the age of 20 are either classified as overweight or obese. Thus, it is an inherent tendency for the majority of individuals to mistakenly select an ineffective method for weight loss. However, intermittent fasting is undeniably one of the most efficacious strategies for achieving weight loss. Multiple studies have extensively demonstrated that regular fasting can considerably aid individuals in reducing their excess body weight. How does this happen?

IF primarily induces ketosis, leading to the creation of a deficit in energy expenditure. In the period of fasting, caloric intake is significantly reduced to near-zero levels while energy expenditure must be maintained at the usual rate. Consequently, without glucose present, the body resorts to utilizing its stored fat reserves and initiates the process of metabolizing them in order to generate energy. When deployed with efficacy, this procedure can function as a harbinger of significant reduction in weight. This mirrors the methodology employed by the "ketogenic diet" in facilitating weight loss. Nevertheless, fasting employs the metabolic state of ketosis in a manner that is both safer and more effortless. The principle of the ketogenic diet revolves around the consumption of high quantities of fats, while simultaneously limiting one's protein and carbohydrate intake. In the practice of intermittent fasting, individuals have the flexibility to consume any desired food during a designated time window, while reallocating the remaining hours for the initiation of the metabolic state known as ketosis. This implies that there is no necessity to deprive your body of essential nutrients.

Lose actual fat

In the realm of IF, individuals are afforded the opportunity to effectively reduce and shed real adipose tissue. How is this so? In order to achieve weight loss, it is essential to maintain a calorie intake level that is lower than the energy expenditure, thereby facilitating the reduction of body weight. IF effectively maximizes this negative equilibrium. Due to your tendency to skip meals, there is a considerable decrease in your calorie consumption. This implies that you can commence the reduction of body fat in a prompt manner. When the act of consuming food occurs after a certain period of time, the probability of consuming a quantity of food that is less than the customary amount is quite high. In the event that, against all odds, you do manage to obtain it, the subsequent fasting cycle will inevitably eradicate the excess.

Planned hormesis

Fasting induces a heightened level of adaptive cellular stress on our cellular components, compelling them to effectively manage a temporary scarcity of essential nutrients. This enhances cellular preparedness to effectively cope with more formidable stressors, such as ailments. This situation exemplifies the well-known adage that adversity can build strength. This principle is commonly referred to as hormesis, and fasting stands out as a highly effective method of activating it.

Mitigates the likelihood of cardiovascular diseases

Intermittent fasting has additionally exhibited the potential to diminish the likelihood of cardiovascular ailments, encompassing conditions like strokes and hypertension. Numerous cardiovascular diseases arise due to the progressive accumulation of lipids along the vasculature. As individuals advance in years, there is a progressive buildup of lipid deposits within our blood vessels, which subsequently undergo oxidation, leading to the formation of arterial plaques. These plaques impede the effective transportation of nutrients across and through the vessels. Indeed, they have the potential to induce a diminished circulation of blood.

IF decreases the likelihood of this occurrence by;

Reducing inflammation and hypertension

Enhancing glucose circulation and lipid profiles Enhancing the circulation of glucose and improving lipid levels

Consequently, numerous research studies have indicated a decrease in LDL cholesterol levels, an increase in HDL cholesterol levels, a reduction in arterial blockages, and a decrease in blood pressure readings among individuals who engage in intermittent fasting. The convergence of these indicators collectively diminishes the probability of experiencing a myocardial infarction or any other ailment pertaining to the cardiovascular system. Furthermore, additional research has demonstrated that individuals adhering to intermittent fasting have exhibited enhanced facilitation of glucose and insulin transfer through vascular linings.

Better sleep

Intermittent fasting additionally fosters advantageous lifestyle adjustments that can support the improvement of your sleep patterns and enhance the level of restfulness you experience. The utilization of Intermittent Fasting assists in averting nocturnal indulgence in food, which may ultimately result in diminished quality of sleep. It is commonsense really. Individuals experience improved sleep quality when they consume a moderate amount of food before bedtime rather than indulging in a large, filling meal.

Increasing cognitive vitality.

If I were to assert that intermittent fasting has the potential to offer superior energy levels compared to a conventional unrestricted diet, one might initially regard this claim as subject to debate. Allow me to provide additional clarification. Lipids and fats have a higher energy yield per calorie compared to glucose. Certainly, you can rely on that assertion. The preference of the body for glucose as its energy substrate does not render it the utmost efficient option available. In addition to this undeniable fact that strongly suggests a heightened energy output with reduced weight, it should be noted that the energy derived from ketosis is noticeably more pristine and devoid of any adverse consequences. When one partakes in a starch-rich meal and as a result, consumes glucose, it leads to a sudden surge and subsequent sharp increase in blood sugar levels. In a brief span, the levels subsequently experience a precipitous decline. This is the elucidation for symptoms such as vertigo and somnolence that occasionally manifest following a substantial meal. When engaging in physical activity while fasting, the energy provided to your body remains pure, untainted by disruptions in sugar levels. The cerebral function is enhanced by the presence of this pristine form of energy.

Effective healing

There exist numerous biological processes within the human body that engender a state of widespread inflammation, with one of such mechanisms being the act of eating. The act of consuming food typically results in insulin secretion and gives rise to systemic inflammation. Hence, when experiencing illness, our body mobilizes all its resources to combat the sickness, leading to a potential decrease in appetite as our body seeks to minimize its exposure to additional sources of inflammation. Fasting however is anti-inflammatory. Indeed, numerous chemical mediators that promote inflammation, such as Interleukin-6, are frequently inhibited during the period of fasting. This implies that reduced inflammation enables your body to undergo more prompt and efficient healing processes.

Autophagy also serves as a significant factor in facilitating the process of healing. Through the acceleration of the repair process of deteriorated tissue, IF facilitates more rapid and enhanced healing.

Favorable alterations in hormone levels Positive shifts in hormone levels Advantageous modifications in hormone levels Profitable adjustments in hormone levels Gainful changes in hormone levels Valuable variations in hormone levels

The investigation of what occurs to human growth hormone during fasting has perpetually been a focal point of scientific inquiry. Human growth hormone (HGH) exerts contrasting effects compared to insulin. While insulin facilitates the transportation of glucose into cells, the role of HGH primarily centers around stimulating the body to enhance its metabolic rate and promote fat reduction. Currently, numerous scientific investigations have corroborated that fasting can lead to a substantial increase in levels of Human Growth Hormone (HGH), reaching up to five times its baseline levels. This results in tangible advantages for the reduction of body fat and the development of muscle mass.

Moreover, this phenomenon is not solely limited to its impact on hormones in a general sense. Insulin, playing a vital role in facilitating glucose utilization, tends to be elevated in individuals who consume a substantial amount of carbohydrates. Over time, the body may develop a reduced sensitivity to circulating insulin due to prolonged exposure to these insulin levels. As a result, in cases where the body fails to properly respond to insulin, there will be a buildup of glucose within the bloodstream. Despite the presence of insulin, glucose uptake into the appropriate cells is impeded due to a lack of recognition by the body towards insulin. This can result in a myriad of health complications. Indeed, this serves as the rationale behind type-2 diabetes. Individuals afflicted with this medical condition possess insulin, yet their physiological systems fail to acknowledge the presence of said insulin. Hence, the entirety of the glucose present in the food they consume is absorbed into their bloodstream, however, it fails to traverse into the cells.

However, with the implementation of intermittent fasting, a paradigm shift occurs. The overall configuration of glucose utilization within the human body undergoes a transformation, instigating various biochemical alterations. Research investigations have demonstrated that individuals who engage in regular fasting generally exhibit reduced insulin levels and experience significant enhancements in insulin sensitivity. Consequently, a reduced amount of insulin is necessary to facilitate the transfer of glucose into the cellular structures. The decreased levels of insulin also facilitate enhanced utilization of stored body fats.

Moreover, intermittent fasting typically alters the hormonal balance within the body, leading to enhanced weight loss during periods of fasting. There will be a discernible decrease in food consumption, coupled with an escalated rate of metabolism. This results in an increased utilization of fat as a primary fuel source during physical activities. In addition to mitigating insulin levels and augmenting growth hormone secretion, fasting also induces an elevation in the quantity of released noradrenaline. Noradrenaline, also referred to as norepinephrine, is a endocrine compound that is synthesized within the adrenal medulla, a glandular structure situated superiorly to the kidneys. In conjunction with its more commonly occurring counterpart, adrenaline, this hormone serves to augment the overall metabolic rate of the body. Accelerated fat oxidation occurs when there is an elevation in noradrenaline levels. In general, fasting has the potential to elevate the overall metabolic rate of the body by a considerable margin of 3.6% to 14%, owing primarily to the hormonal fluctuations that occur during this period. That is right. The body must adapt to a new energy source and resorts to consuming fast-burning fuels as the resolution.

Enhanced cognitive abilities and improved memory capacity

Given that individuals adhering to an Intermittent Fasting regimen generally exhibit elevated levels of BDNF, a discernible relationship can be observed between IF and enhancements in cognitive capacities and mental acuity. According to the literature by Michael VanDerschelden titled "The Scientific Approach to Intermittent Fasting," it has been demonstrated that intermittent fasting induces a noteworthy elevation of BDNF levels ranging from 50 to 400 percent, depending on the particular cerebral region under consideration. The neurons within the human body transmit signals to the brain and convey instructions to all other regions of the body. By fostering the preservation of neuronal integrity and promoting overall brain health, the decision to adhere to an intermittent fasting regimen can substantially enhance cognitive abilities.

Exercise and Fasting

Engaging in physical activity is regarded as one of the most beneficial pursuits in terms of improving overall well-being for individuals. "It offers a plethora of health advantages such as;

Reduces the levels of glucose in the bloodstream

Increases insulin sensitivity

Facilitates the process of lipolysis (the hydrolysis and subsequent mobilization of lipids)

Increases growth hormone

These advantages represent just a fraction of the total range of benefits it offers. The advantages are further amplified when physical activity coincides with fasting. Despite the potential challenge of reduced endurance caused by hunger, engaging in exercise during a fasting state can yield twice the customary advantages. Nonetheless, what if I were to inform you that intermittent fasting not only enhances these advantages of physical activity, but also generates them independently. Intermittent fasting (IF) serves as a type of metabolic exercise that enhances the body's capacity to endure challenging conditions, regenerate its own tissues, and purify all the physiological systems within.

Intermittent fasting confers an extensive array of health advantages for individuals of all backgrounds. There exist a plethora of additional examples, which exceed the capacity to be addressed within the confines of this literary work.

Intermittent Fasting Protocol: Eat-Stop-Eat

This protocol is well-suited for individuals who already maintain a nutritious diet and are seeking to augment their health regimen. The primary focus of the Eat-Stop-Eat (referred to as ESE for conciseness) protocol lies in practicing moderation. You are permitted to consume a wide range of foods, provided they are consumed in moderate portions. Want to eat cake? Please feel free to indulge in a single slice, but please refrain from consuming the entire cake. Want a donut? Enjoy one but not the whole box.

How to practice

It is undeniably the most straightforward among the protocols as it entails fasting only once or twice a week – no more, no less! During these fasting periods, you are unrestricted in your food choices. Nevertheless, it is imperative that each fast extends for a continuous period of 24 hours. And that is the primary area where individuals typically encounter the greatest level of difficulty. You are permitted to consume an unrestricted amount of calorie-free beverages on the fasting days. Following the completion of your 24-hour fast, simply resume consuming meals in a moderate manner.

The determination of the optimal timing and duration for your fasts throughout the week is entirely at your discretion. You may duly consider your personal schedule and social commitments in order to minimize any inconvenience and ensure adherence to the proposed plan. Adhering to this fasting approach will enable you to reduce your overall weekly caloric intake without enduring daily hardship. Just like any other reputable and efficacious weight loss protocols, the incorporation of regular physical activity is essential to optimize the weight reduction advantages achievable through this program. More specifically, it is imperative that you give precedence to weightlifting exercises. However, if it is unattainable to engage in those activities, any form of regular exercise will suffice, such as brisk walking or cycling, although the enhancement in weight loss may not be as substantial as that observed with weightlifting.

Advantages

Notwithstanding the extended duration of the 24-hour fasting period, this protocol demonstrates remarkable adaptability. Especially in the initial stages, it is not necessary to fully commit oneself, that is, to forgo nourishment for the entire duration of 24 hours. On the initial fasting days, endeavor to abstain from consuming any food for as long as possible, gradually extending the duration until you can effectively observe a 24-hour fast on your selected day or days of the week. It is advisable to commence the fast during a time of high productivity, as one's mind will be engrossed in tasks, offering a diversion from hunger and reducing its conscious perception, in contrast to periods of idleness.

Another benefit is that there are a limited number of forbidden foods and there is no requirement to meticulously track one's caloric consumption. As previously stated, the crucial factor at hand is moderation, thus the sole recommendation pertaining to consumption is to maintain moderate serving sizes. feeling too deprived to afterwards is quite low. Therefore, the probability of reaching the state of binge-eating is increased.

Another evident advantage of this protocol is the decrease in caloric intake, which is beneficial for achieving effective weight loss. You'll be able to significantly cut down on calories not on a daily basis, which may be hard especially if you're busy, but on a weekly basis. Within a mere span of 48 hours, it is within your grasp to attain the necessary reduction in calorie intake for the entirety of the week. Consequently, you will only be compelled to abstain from consuming food for a maximum of two instances per week, with each fasting period extending over a duration of 24 hours. If you are able to consistently adhere to this approach, which is highly likely given the straightforward nature of the protocol, you should be capable of attaining your desired body weight or composition expeditiously, particularly when complemented by a regimen of regular weightlifting exercises.

In addition to the ESE protocol, one can also expect to experience improved insulin sensitivity and increased levels of growth hormone, which are both advantageous outcomes. As previously stated, a decrease in food consumption consequently leads to a decrease in the production of insulin by the body. In such instances, the body exhibits heightened responsiveness to insulin, a crucial element in facilitating successful weight reduction, specifically in terms of fat loss.

Growth hormones play a crucial role in stimulating and enhancing the body's fat-burning capacities, primarily by promoting the preservation or augmentation of muscle mass. Growth hormone production reaches its optimal levels exclusively at three distinct times throughout the day: during or immediately following sleep, immediately after engaging in vigorous exercise for a minimum duration of 10 minutes, and shortly after concluding the period of fasting. This indicates that sustained release of growth hormone occurs during sleep and extended exercise durations of over 10 minutes. By adopting a pattern of fasting for two full days per week, extending for a duration of 24 hours each time, your body's production of growth hormone can be further enhanced during the intervals when you discontinue these fasting periods. Consequently, this heightened production of growth hormone holds significant implications. Indeed, achieving the ideal fat reduction!

Disadvantages

The sole drawback of this protocol pertains to the duration of fasting that it necessitates. An infrequent period of 24-hour fasting should not be taken lightly. Additionally, if you plan to engage in this activity on a regular basis, specifically at least twice per week.

It is highly probable that achieving complete implementation, especially within the initial days or weeks, is an exceedingly challenging endeavor. A potential approach to address this issue is to commence from your current starting point, that is to say, refraining from eating for as long as possible within a 24-hour timeframe, and progressively extending the duration of fasting until you are eventually capable of consistently fasting for 24 hours consecutively.

The Significance of the Fuel We Utilize

Some nutrition basics

While it is unnecessary to follow any specific "diet" while practicing intermittent fasting, it is important to consider a few key factors. Please be aware that processed food should never be considered as a beneficial companion. If you possess a comprehensive understanding of nutrition, you may choose to omit this portion if you wish. If you lack certainty or are not entirely confident, let us acquire some simple strategies to enhance our proficiency.

In order to prioritize our well-being, optimize our digestive function, and enhance our overall nutritional intake, it is imperative that we refrain from consuming excessively processed food items. To simplify the task, it is advisable to adhere to the consumption of meat, produce, and grains. Please refrain from consuming pre-packaged snacks and meals to the greatest extent possible. When engaging in grocery shopping, it is advisable to confine oneself to the periphery of the store rather than venturing into the interior aisles. Make an effort to primarily patronize farmers markets or food cooperatives whenever feasible. It is important to bear in mind that adhering to an eating window of 8 hours allows us to consume a reduced number of meals, thereby enabling us to allocate our resources towards purchasing high-quality, nutrient-rich products.

If you are purchasing commercially prepared food items, please examine the packaging. Please refrain from purchasing food items that contain hydrogenated substances or high fructose corn syrup. Refrain from purchasing any products containing a compilation of ingredients that are not comprehensible to you. Endeavor to exclusively purchase food products composed solely of natural ingredients. Prepackaged food may be acceptable, provided that it is devoid of any additives or elements commonly associated with processed food. Your physique is incapable of making any use of such substances. It merely serves to obstruct and impede the efficient functioning of the elegant system.

Macronutrients

Our cuisine consists of three essential macronutrients, namely: fat, carbohydrate, and protein. Every individual bears a highly distinct and specialized function within the human anatomy. While our objective through intermittent fasting is not centered around imposing restrictions on ourselves, akin to a conventional diet, acquiring knowledge about our essential macronutrients can aid us in making more informed and judicious choices.

Allow us to engage in a discussion surrounding two of our most commonly misinterpreted foundational elements. Fats and carbohydrates merit significantly more acknowledgement than we typically confer upon them.

Fat

In a bygone era, as you may recollect, fat was vilified. We attributed all possible maladies within ourselves to it, and instead of adopting a healthier diet, we opted to eliminate fat from all aspects of our food. Quite literally, we have considered every conceivable possibility. We successfully implemented fat reduction in a wide range of products, including snacks, crackers, desserts, cookies, candy bars, and bread. Our comprehensive approach targeted the removal of fats from various food items, reflecting our commitment to delivering healthier options to consumers. But fat carries flavor. It enhances the flavor of food. Without the presence of fats, we are left with a culinary product that has the unpleasant taste and texture resembling that of cardboard. In order to enhance its taste, we incorporated sweeteners. We utilized a variety of sugars, including real sugar, artificial sweeteners, and corn-based sweeteners, effectively incorporating them into our products.

And individuals experienced a sense of contentment as they were able to consume an entire package of low-fat cheese crackers, all the while maintaining a positive perception of their own well-being. They could substitute their regular choices with fat-free alternatives, consume a greater quantity than before, while simultaneously experiencing a sense of satisfaction in their healthy eating habits, without feeling as if they were depriving themselves or deviating from their dietary goals, thus resulting in increased food consumption. We indulged in an excessive consumption of unhealthy, refined carbohydrates, resulting in unfavorable outcomes of increased size and deteriorating health.

However, the issue at hand was never specifically related to excess body weight. It was consistently the latent undesirable carbohydrates, and we exacerbated the situation. It is a fact that we require fat in our bodies. We require it for virtually every physiological process, with the utmost significance being attributed to hormone synthesis. Our hormones permeate our bodies, enabling the operations of every routine mechanism. All biological processes, including concentration, physical exertion, sexual reproduction, and general sexual activity, as well as energy regulation, reading, speaking, and every single action we undertake, are all facilitated by the influence of hormones within our bodies.

When there is a dysfunction in our hormonal balance, our overall well-being is compromised. They bear a significant amount of responsibility for both our physical and mental well-being. Fat is essential in aiding the synthesis of our body's hormones.

Of comparable significance is the role fat assumes in both brain function and the regulation of inflammation. Fat is necessary for maintaining the health of the skin, insulation, safeguarding organs, as well as providing overall energy.

139

Naturally, not all fats possess identical characteristics. Foods such as olive oil, nuts, seeds, avocados, and fish are rich in beneficial, unsaturated fats. These fatty substances contribute to enhancing your overall quality of life, promoting a higher level of comfort, and mitigating the occurrence of inflammatory responses. These polyunsaturated fats play a vital role in maintaining a well-balanced dietary regimen. Let us consider them as our utmost coveted adipose tissue.

However, one must consider the impact of saturated fats. Although it may appear paradoxical, the presence of saturated fats and cholesterol in our diet plays a crucial role in facilitating the production of testosterone and human growth hormone within our bodies. One aspect of the intermittent fasting experience that brings great satisfaction is the capacity to preserve and promote muscle development as opposed to diminishing it, all the while engaging in the process of fat burning. To optimize the benefits derived from this lifestyle, it is imperative to include a moderate amount of saturated fat on a daily basis. It is not an aspect to which we wish to excessively dedicate our efforts. Eggs, butter, and coconut oil are all viable alternatives, wherein eggs possess the additional advantage of being rich in favorable cholesterol. However, it must be acknowledged that certain types of saturated fats possess beneficial properties, while others have been artificially produced and are considered highly detrimental. Let's discuss.

Fats to avoid. Certain types of fats can be considered detrimental to one's health. Poor quality fats have undergone extensive refinement, resulting in their transformation into substances with carcinogenic properties. In essence, they will gradually cause your demise whilst maintaining everlasting life. That is their point. Hydrogenated oil, also known as trans fats, possess exceptional stability and can endure extensive periods without spoiling.

Hydrogenated oils denote vegetable oils that have undergone chemical modification to inhibit food spoilage, thereby enhancing food preservation and cost efficiency for manufacturers. The hydrogenation process entails the incorporation of hydrogen atoms into the existing double bonds present in the oil. As the degree of hydrogenation rises, the content of saturated fat becomes elevated while the content of unsaturated fat diminishes.

When incorporated into a baked product, they exhibit a long shelf life of at least 6 months. It is commonly believed that Twinkies and cockroaches possess the remarkable ability to endure even when all other forms of life have perished. That's the hydrogenated oil. In the event that a zombie apocalypse engulfs the planet, kindly indulge in those decadently delectable cakes that remain freshly baked. The possibility exists that the zombies could apprehend you prior to the disease having an opportunity. However, in the contemporary world, perhaps the most benevolent action you can take for your own well-being is to refrain from consuming hydrogenated oils.

The issue with trans fats, also known as hydrogenated oil, lies in their tendency to essentially counteract all the objectives we seek to accomplish. They elevate LDL cholesterol levels while reducing HDL cholesterol levels. They inhibit the synthesis of substances that counteract inflammation and confer advantages to the endocrine and neurological systems, concurrently permitting the presence of substances that promote inflammation. As a result, trans fats tend to induce inflammation and adversely affect cholesterol levels, rather than reducing inflammation and promoting hormonal balance, which is characteristic of our beneficial unsaturated fats. They embody wickedness in the delectable guise of miniature chocolate donuts.

To evade the presence of hydrogenated oils, it is imperative to diligently examine both the nutritional information and ingredients listed on product labels. Numerous food products that are marketed as having "zero grams of trans fat" actually contain trans fat.

In accordance with the guidelines outlined by the FDA, if the quantity of trans fat per serving is lower than 0.5 grams, the manufacturer is permitted to indicate "zero grams trans fat" on the nutrition label.

This is where the practice of scrutinizing ingredients becomes essential. If the list of ingredients includes the terms "hydrogenated" or "partially hydrogenated," it can be concluded that the food product contains trans fat. Once more, some of the numerous reprocessed food items known to contain trans fats encompass baked goods, snack items, foods subjected to deep-frying, and certain margarine products. Whenever feasible, it is advised to prepare one's own meals rather than purchasing prepackaged options.

Carbohydrates

Carbohydrates can be regarded as a relatively more recent adversary when compared to fats. Similar to dietary fats, carbohydrates are essential and often subject to misconceptions.

Carbohydrates play a pivotal role as the primary and essential source of energy for the human body. The human body has the ability to promptly utilize these substances, alternatively, they can be stored within the liver and muscles for future utilization.

Consuming carbohydrates is a vital component of maintaining a well-balanced and nutritious dietary regimen. However, it is crucial to acquire knowledge on the types and proportions of carbohydrates that are suitable for consumption, as not all carbohydrates possess the same nutritional value.

Strive to consume carbohydrates that are rich in nutritional content. Direct your attention towards complex carbohydrates that possess a significant fiber content, denoting a minimum of 5 grams per serving. They will afford you a prolonged sensation of satisfaction while minimizing caloric intake. The crux of the matter lies in opting for unprocessed, whole foods over their processed counterparts. Fruits and numerous vegetables are abundant in carbohydrates. In addition to harnessing clean energy, you are also benefiting from the ingestion of fiber, vitamins, and minerals. You are effectively fostering significant benefits for your physical well-being without imposing any additional strain on the elimination or management of any potentially detrimental substances or excessive elements. Dairy is an additional source of carbohydrates that provides an abundance of additional nutrients, such as protein.

Protein

Protein is renowned for its significance in muscle development, which aligns precisely with our objective of maintaining strength and a toned physique (it is crucial to note that muscles also contribute to heightened caloric expenditure). However, the role of protein extends beyond this aspect. Protein plays a crucial role in various physiological processes such as cellular repair and regeneration, oxygen transportation across the body, bolstering immune function, among other important functions.

Proteins, composed of amino acids, play a vital role in maintaining optimal bodily functions. It constitutes a significant aspect of our identity, playing a pivotal role in nearly all our endeavors.

Animal-based food products, including meat, fish, poultry, dairy, and eggs, possess a comprehensive range of proteins, thereby displaying a harmonious distribution of the 9 fundamental amino acids that are crucial for the human body and readily accessible for optimal utilization. Quinoa, soybeans, and chia seeds are among the limited non-animal sources that provide a complete protein profile.

How to consume according to your dietary requirements

Each of the macronutrients fulfills a crucial function within the human body. Living would be extremely challenging if any one of them were absent. Although strategies such as the elimination of carbohydrates may yield short-term results, it is imperative to maintain a well-rounded dietary intake in order to ensure optimal bodily functions in the long run.

Regarding the precise details of your dietary intake, it is essential to recognize that every individual possesses a distinct and advanced gut microbiome. The intricacies and distinctiveness of our physical beings are notable. What is effective in terms of dietary preferences for one individual may not necessarily yield the same results for another. If individuals perceive unfavorable bodily responses to certain substances, it is expedient to contemplate the implementation of a short-term elimination diet to identify and address the specific food item causing the issue, thereby facilitating further progress in managing the condition. Despite not having any specific food sensitivities, certain individuals perform optimally when their diet contains a higher proportion of carbohydrates. Certain individuals experience optimal well-being by consuming predominantly meat, while there are those who completely eliminate it from their diets. If you opt to exclude meat from your diet, please exercise caution. Please be mindful that your body still requires essential proteins, which are abundantly present in eggs, dairy products, and select plant-based foods. Frequently, individuals may be inclined to excessively depend on carbohydrates when abstaining from meat, thereby giving rise to potential complications. One should bear in mind that maintaining a state of equilibrium is crucial, and it is imperative to discover and achieve such equilibrium that best suits one's own unique physical constitution.

It is crucial to maintain a cognizance of one's food and beverage consumption. This will facilitate the identification of the most optimal course of action tailored to oneself, thereby fostering a heightened rapport with one's own body. Do not lend credence to the exaggerated claims surrounding any novel dietary regimen without conducting thorough research. It is imperative for one to have insight into how their own body responds prior to undertaking any radical measures.

If you are consuming your meals in a manner that provides you with a predominantly positive experience, you may continue to adhere to this pattern while undertaking the process of fasting. If you opt to exclude dairy, meat, simple carbohydrates, or any other food groups, it is perfectly acceptable (however, it is important to consider the essential macronutrients your body requires). Even if you ascertain a preference for consuming solely unhealthy foods, it is deemed acceptable. From a medical standpoint, I do not mean this in terms of one's well-being. And it is highly advised against... however, it is likely within your capabilities. It is highly likely that you will still experience a decrease in weight.

The inherent attractiveness of intermittent fasting lies in... It is 100% personalized. It constitutes a modification in conduct rather than any kind of dietary regimen. And it works wonders.

While it is within your prerogative to engage in intermittent fasting using your preferred method, it is crucial to acknowledge that prioritizing a clean diet, free of processed foods, will invariably be advantageous to your overall well-being. A significant aspect of the intermittent fasting regimen is experiencing improved well-being. During the process of fasting, the body reallocates the energy typically utilized for digestion towards the tasks of cleansing and repairing. The task of facilitating recovery becomes significantly more manageable when one does not have to eliminate unwanted substances and toxins from the body.

Enhances The Functionality Of The Immune System While Aiding In The Process Of Cancer Recuperation.

Fasting is an effective means of initiating a boost to one's immune system. Intermittent fasting stimulates the generation of fresh white blood cells within the body, thus replenishing one's system with active agents that combat diseases. Fasting effectively stimulates the resetting of your immune system, leading to a revitalized immune response.

Especially in the context of a compromised immune system, the periodicity of fasting can facilitate the development of a rejuvenated immune system. Cancer patients generally exhibit diminished immune functions, necessitating the use of medication designed to enhance their immune response.

Upon initiation of fasting, an assortment of white blood cells within the organism is diminished, thereby instigating alterations that facilitate the generation and rejuvenation of nascent immunological cells stemming from stem cells. To be more precise, there is a decrease in the activity of the enzyme PKA, thus inhibiting the specific gene that needs to be suppressed for these stem cells to enter regenerative mode. It effectively signals the activation of stem cells to initiate a process of cell division and regeneration, leading to the restoration of the entire system.

Additional advantages of intermittent fasting encompass:

Boosting metabolism

Preventing inflammation

Improving mood

Slows down aging

Enhances the overall well-being of your skin.

Encourages expedited healing following injury

Having acquired a comprehension of the multitude of advantages associated with intermittent fasting, let us now divert our attention towards examining the diverse array of intermittent fasting approaches that one can embrace in order to shed pounds and successfully attain their weight loss objectives.

Guidelines for Embracing Intermittent Fasting

The initial phase of commencing intermittent fasting involves the selection of an appropriate intermittent fasting technique. In this segment, we will examine the prevailing intermittent fasting techniques, encompassing their advantages and disadvantages, in order for you to make a well-informed decision.

The 5:2 Plan

This approach is widely implemented within the field of IF. Michael Mosley, a healthcare professional and esteemed British journalist, played a key role in its popularization.

According to the 5:2 dietary regimen, individuals are required to limit their caloric intake to approximately 600 calories for men and 500 calories for women on two separate non-consecutive days each week. Following the two-day fasting period, you may resume regular eating habits for the remaining five days, while avoiding the feeling of being constrained by a restrictive diet. This implies that during the days of fasting, you are permitted to consume three meals, albeit in considerably reduced portions. It is frequently suggested that individuals consume one or two meals as an alternative approach to adhere to the calorie limitation.

The 5:2 plan can facilitate the reduction of stored body fat by maintaining a calorie deficit throughout the week. If one is accustomed to consuming 1,600 calories on a daily basis, they will be lowering their overall calorie intake by 2,200 calories. This elucidates the reason behind the assertion that individuals following the 5:2 plan typically experience a weekly reduction of approximately 0.5 to 2 pounds, contingent upon their initial weight.

Pros

The plan does not impose any rigorous dietary limitations on your regular days, affording you the freedom to choose your fasting days based on your personal schedule. In the event that you have a scheduled dinner function or party, it is possible to arrange your meals in such a manner that you designate your fast days on the remaining days, offering flexibility to vary them on a week-to-week basis.

Certain individuals actually favor the 5:2 regimen as it solely necessitates the monitoring and limitation of dietary intake on two specific occasions each week, thereby allowing indulgence in preferred food choices for the remainder of the week. This facilitates the process by providing an accessible and enduring strategy for lifelong implementation.

The cons

A significant issue with this plan lies in its lack of consistency. Given that a daily fasting routine is not followed, adjusting to this schedule may prove challenging and result in excessive hunger on fasting days. Furthermore, a daily intake of only 500 calories is particularly minimal, especially for individuals accustomed to consuming approximately 2000 calories or more on a daily basis. This implies that those particular days can prove to be challenging, especially if you are also partaking in physical activities, performing laborious tasks, or have familial duties (where you must endeavor to disregard the consumption of food by others).

As one might surmise, it is possible to consume excessive amounts of food on the day following a period of fasting, which could potentially impede progress towards weight loss.

Chapter 3: Practical Issues

You now possess a rudimentary understanding of the physiological impact of fasting on your body. It would be advantageous to consider the present moment as an opportune occasion to examine the methods and suitability of various fasting techniques with respect to your individual requirements. It is of utmost importance to comprehend that there exists a substantial disparity between fasting and starving. Fasting constitutes a conscious decision to refrain from consuming nourishment for a prearranged duration, whereas starvation arises from an inadvertent deprivation of sustenance.

It is imperative to comprehend that there are no rigid guidelines dictating the manner or timing of fasting. We will examine several commonly utilized approaches individuals employ when integrating fasting into their lifestyles, allowing you to personalize and adapt these methods according to your specific needs. It is imperative, however, that you possess a comprehensive understanding of the principles and motivations underlying these strategies.

It has been demonstrated previously that the metabolic process of burning the glucose present in your bloodstream requires a duration exceeding sixteen hours. Subsequently, you will initiate the process of fat oxidation, whereby the duration of your fasting period directly correlates with the extent of fat combustion. Although some individuals may prefer to begin with a prolonged, intensive fast, it is perhaps more pragmatic to integrate a sequence of shorter yet consistent fasts into one's routine, thereby establishing a habitual practice rather than engaging in a temporary and restrictive diet trend.

A method to accomplish this goal is by engaging in fasts lasting for a period of sixteen hours. The majority of individuals have a tendency to abstain from eating during the period between dinner and breakfast. By refraining from consuming any food after 8 p.m. and until noon the next day, you will provide ample opportunity for your body to metabolize a substantial portion of the glucose present in your bloodstream. This represents a straightforward and relatively painless method of fasting, whereby if one avoids excessive consumption upon reinitiating the intake of food, gradual experiencing of health benefits can be anticipated from this approach alone. It is likely that you have been taught to regard breakfast as the most crucial meal of the day. However, there is a dearth of significant scientific evidence supporting this belief, and much of the existing evidence has been funded by prominent cereal manufacturers. Although there may be some advantages to this type of fasting, it is improbable that significant weight loss will occur as your body is not compelled to engage in fat burning for a substantial period of time.

A more rigorous form of fasting is referred to as the 5:2 protocol, which entails adhering to a regular eating pattern for five days in a week, whereas abstaining from food for two periods lasting twenty four hours each within that same week. Should one consume a regular amount of food on Monday and subsequently refrain from eating until dinner on Tuesday, they would have effectively completed a twenty-four hour fast. By engaging in this pattern of rapid repetition later in the week, you are adhering to the 5:2 fasting protocol. The majority of individuals on this system strive to consume no more than six hundred calories during the initial meal following the fasting period. Your body will have undergone two consecutive periods of twenty-four hours during the week, in which it entered a ketogenic state. This lifestyle approach is highly sustainable and expected to yield significant weight loss results, as long as you refrain from indulging excessively on non-fasting days. In addition, it intertwines seamlessly with the practice of a sixteen-hour daily fasting regimen, which involves omitting breakfast, making the amalgamation of these fasting approaches widely favored. The decrease is substantially significant in terms of calorie content. Assuming your regular daily calorie intake is 2000 calories, your cumulative calorie consumption over the course of a week would amount to 14000 calories. Two days a week you are knocking that intake down to just 600 calories per day which gives you a weekly reduction of 2800 calories. This yields a monthly calorie deficit of 11200 calories, representing a significant cost reduction. Considering that once you acclimate to this dietary regimen, it has the potential to evolve into a continual and viable way of life, it becomes apparent how this fasting method can effectively facilitate weight reduction while concurrently decreasing glucose and insulin levels in the bloodstream.

Certain individuals opt for observing a period of fasting spanning only a single day per week, while others prefer to undertake a more prolonged fast occurring just once within a month. The potential combinations are vast, yet it is advisable to exercise sound judgment. Your objective should focus on the establishment of a durable and sustainable dietary approach that facilitates gradual weight reduction. Pursuing drastic crash diets for weight loss is neither conducive to one's overall wellbeing nor can it be maintained in the long term. It is advisable to maintain regular intake of fluids such as water or green teas, and not solely rely on thirst as an indicator of hydration. The consumption of beverages can facilitate the removal of accumulated toxins from the body, thereby providing an supplementary advantage for overall well-being.

It is crucial to cultivate the habit of consuming food solely when experiencing genuine hunger. Our species has undergone adaptation to endure periods of both abundance and scarcity; however, we find ourselves currently existing in a prolonged period of perpetual surplus. This is a cultivated behavior for which our physical organisms have not adequately adjusted. Therefore, it is necessary to acquaint oneself with the capacity to discern genuine hunger prior to commencing a meal. The conventional practice of consuming three daily meals deviates from natural behavior, and once one adjusts to consuming smaller portions, they often discover the ability to skip meals due to decreased need. The act of consuming food should no longer be established as a customary practice.

Chapter Three: Identifying Optimal Approaches

There exist several intermittent fasting approaches that one can contemplate. Given that intermittent fasting can be customized to accommodate any schedule of your choice, you are presented with the opportunity to select a technique that is most suitable for your individual circumstances. Regardless of the approach you opt for, you can be assured of accomplishing your objectives pertaining to weight loss, physical fitness, and overall well-being.

It is imperative to acknowledge that the methodology one selects may yield superior outcomes compared to those of others, and vice versa. If one genuinely desires to adopt intermittent fasting as a sustained way of life, it is advisable to experiment with various approaches and ultimately choose the one that aligns most harmoniously with their individual lifestyle.

Approaches to Intermittent Fasting

1. The Leangains Protocol" could be rephrased as "The Leangains Protocol is outlined.

This particular fasting approach is widely recognized as one of the most popular methods for intermittent fasting, commonly referred to as the 16/8 method. It entails abstaining from food intake for a duration of 14 to 16 hours on a daily basis. Consequently, the consumption period is limited to a span of 8 to 10 hours per day. While to some, this duration may appear relatively brief, employing this approach enables individuals to consume approximately two to three meals within this specific time frame.

The Leangains approach is, in fact, remarkably uncomplicated. One can opt to abstain from consuming any form of dessert following the evening meal, consequently forgoing breakfast the next morning. While asleep, you will essentially be engaging in a fasting state. If you partook in an evening repast at 8 o'clock, it is recommended that your subsequent meal be scheduled approximately at noon the following day. Consequently, you will have refrained from eating for a total duration of 16 hours. Within the fasting period, you are authorized to drink water and non-alcoholic beverages. Nevertheless, it is essential to adhere to a diet consisting of nutritious foods that are unrefined and devoid of processing, exclusively within the designated 8-hour period designated for eating.

The Leangains approach is tailored to individuals who engage in regular exercise with the intention of shedding weight and enhancing muscle tone. On days when engaging in physical activity, it is advisable to prioritize the consumption of carbohydrates over fats. During days of rest, it is advised to consume a greater proportion of dietary fats compared to carbohydrates. Maintain a consistently elevated intake of protein throughout, taking into account factors such as age, gender, and levels of physical activity. The temporal gaps between meals do not hold significant importance, allowing for flexibility in determining when to eat. However, it is widely acknowledged that dividing the feeding window into three distinct meals is a more convenient approach for many individuals. Nevertheless, this approach exhibits a high degree of inflexibility when it comes to defining the specific dietary choices, particularly for individuals engaged in physical exercise.

This approach typically suggests that women observe a fasting period of 14 hours, while men adhere to a complete fasting period of 16 hours. This trend can be attributed to the fact that women tend to exhibit superior performance during shorter, rapid intervals. Additionally, maintaining a consistent eating window is of utmost importance, as any deviation may significantly disrupt hormonal balance and overall bodily function.

2. The method known as the 5:2 Diet

This method involves eating normally for 5 days in a week and then cutting down your calorie intake for the remaining two days of the week. This approach is commonly known as the Fast Diet. It is advised that women restrict their calorie intake to 500 on fasting days, while men should limit their calorie intake to 600.

You are granted the autonomy to select the two weekdays in which you are most inclined to observe abstinence or fasting. During these specific days, it is obligatory for you to partake in two modest-sized meals, wherein each meal should consist of either 250 calories for women or 300 calories for men.

Detractors of this approach contend that the diet in question has yet to undergo empirical scrutiny, although they do concur with the notion that intermittent fasting, as a whole, yields numerous advantages.

3. The method of intermittent fasting known as the 'Eat-Stop-Eat' protocol

This fast is performed on a weekly basis, either once or twice, lasting for a duration of 24 hours. This approach is equally well-received and is tailored to individuals who have a preference for maintaining a nutritious diet and are in pursuit of an additional source of energy.

You have the option to decide on your preferred method of fasting for the duration of 24 hours. As an illustration, one can partake in dinner at 8 pm and subsequently observe an interval until 8 pm on the ensuing day before consuming the subsequent meal. If it so happens that your inclination leans towards having breakfast or lunch, it will be requisite for you to abstain from food until the subsequent breakfast or lunch. Please endeavor to allocate it within your timetable. The selection of meals one chooses to forgo holds no significance, as the fasting period spans a full 24 hours.

It is imperative that you refrain from ingesting solid food during the fasting period. Your intake should solely consist of water and non-alcoholic beverages. If your goal is weight reduction, ensure that your dietary habits remain unchanged during your designated eating period. Stated differently, once the period of fasting concludes, it is recommended to consume meals as if abstaining from fasting had not been practiced at all. This approach is most effective when supplemented with resistance training to facilitate greater weight loss and optimize muscle growth.

This approach may pose considerable challenges for novices due to the demanding nature of abstaining from food for an entire 24-hour period. It is advisable to commence with a fasting period of 14 hours and gradually extend it. Adherence to discipline is an essential element within this approach.

The advantages of this approach lie in its inherent flexibility, absence of the need for caloric calculations, and lack of constraints regarding food choices.

4. The Regimen of Alternate-Day Fasting

This approach is commonly known as the UpDayDownDay Diet and is specifically tailored for conscientious individuals pursuing their desired weight loss goals. This dietary approach entails a period of severe calorie restriction followed by a return to regular eating habits on the subsequent day.

During the days designated for fasting (commonly known as Down Days), it is advisable to restrict your caloric consumption to approximately one-fifth of your normal intake. It is advisable to opt for replacement shakes over solid foods, as they come preloaded with vital nutrients that can be consumed gradually throughout the day. This approach ought to be implemented solely during the initial fortnight, subsequent to which, it is advisable to return to the consumption of solid sustenance.

You are strongly encouraged to reserve your strenuous workout sessions for your regular eating days, also known as Up Days. This approach presents a straightforward implementation, albeit necessitating caution to prevent indulging excessively during Up Days. In order to circumvent this issue, it is crucial to meticulously strategize and arrange your meals beforehand.

5. The Warrior Diet regimen

This approach entails the consumption of small portions of fruits and vegetables throughout the day, followed by the ingestion of a substantial meal during the evening. You are essentially adhering to a dietary pattern that involves abstaining from food consumption throughout the day, and subsequently consuming meals only within a limited 4-hour timeframe in the evening. It can be confidently stated that the Warrior diet is well-suited for individuals displaying a high level of self-discipline.

The diet you adhere to should consist of Paleo-compliant ingredients that are in their whole and unaltered state. This approach is grounded in the belief that human beings are nocturnal eaters and that the intake of nutrients should align with our circadian rhythms. Through the consumption of minute portions of fruits, vegetables, or protein throughout the day, one's nervous system is enlivened, energy levels are heightened, and the stimulation of fat-burning is facilitated. Consuming excessive amounts of food during the evening hours contributes to the restoration of the nervous system, facilitates tranquility, and improves the process of digestion.

This approach exhibits a stringent adherence to the prescribed sequence for food consumption. During the allotted period of four hours designated for meals, it is customary to consume vegetables initially, followed by subsequent intake of proteins and fats. If you still find yourself hungry, it would be advisable to consume some carbohydrates.

Advocates of this approach assert that they observe heightened energy levels and a reduction in adipose tissue. The permissibility of consuming food during daylight hours contributes to its widespread popularity. Nevertheless, it is challenging to sustain this approach as a permanent lifestyle. The stringent meal plan might have an impact on your social interactions, as it is uncommon for individuals to consume large meals in the evening.

6. Permanently Achieving Weight Loss

This amalgamation comprises elements from the Warrior Diet, Eat-Stop-Eat, and Leangains. It comprises a structured regimen and instructional regimen wherein one abstains from food and undergoes a continuous fasting period of 36 hours, followed by the allocation of the remaining days of the week to the three different fasting techniques. An advantage is that you have the privilege of having one day each week to indulge.

The aforementioned program was devised by individuals named Dan Go and John Romaniello. They offer the fasting regimen through the official website www.fatlossforever.net. Additionally, the plan incorporates exercises that involve the use of weights and exercises that utilize one's own body weight.

One issue associated with this plan is the necessity of maintaining self-restraint in order to avoid excessive indulgence during designated cheat days. The plan is equally perplexing due to its inflexibility combined with the fluctuating schedule. Conversely, you will receive a personalized calendar that complements the program, thereby enhancing its manageability.

Food for Thought

The aforementioned six techniques represent the most widely recognized approaches to intermittent fasting. There exist alternative options that demonstrate greater adaptability. It is important to acknowledge that fasting may not be suitable for every individual. The methodologies exhibit unique qualities due to the disparate protocols which necessitate compliance. It is recommended that you seek guidance from your healthcare provider prior to beginning any fasting regimen. Certain individuals may be exempt from fasting due to underlying medical conditions, therefore it is crucial to carefully consider all relevant factors before making a decision regarding the preferred approach.

Approach 2: The Intermittent Fasting Every Other Day Method

Moving forward, we shall now delve into an additional approach known as alternate day fasting. An alternative way to express the same information in a formal tone could be: "This method can also be referred to as the 'Up Day Down Day diet,' which was introduced by the renowned fitness expert, Dr. James Johnson."

How does it work?

Similar to any other methodology, the underlying concept is equally straightforward. You engage in a cyclic pattern of alternating between days of fasting and days of not fasting. This signifies that in the event that you consume a regular amount of food today, you will abstain from eating the following day, and resume your regular eating pattern on the subsequent day. You merely adhere to that sequence on alternate days throughout the week.

Nonetheless, employing this approach does not entail engaging in full-day fasting. On your fasting days, it is indeed possible to consume one-fifth of your typical calorie intake. Stated differently, should one consume a daily caloric intake ranging from 2000 to 2500 calories, it is advisable to decrease the amount to approximately 400 to 500 calories during fasting days.

For whom is it most suitable?

Undoubtedly, this approach may not be universally suitable for all individuals. For example, individuals who are new to intermittent fasting may encounter challenges in adopting this approach due to the extended duration of fasting.

This approach is particularly suitable for individuals who possess strong self-discipline and are driven by a clear and specific weight objective.

Consider the following perspective: do you possess the necessary level of discipline to meticulously monitor your calorie intake for each meal amid your fasting periods? For the majority of individuals, this may appear to entail an excessive amount of effort. If such an impression resonates with you, it may be advisable to explore an alternate intermittent fasting approach.

How to do it

"If after conducting a thorough self-assessment, you have made the informed decision to embrace this approach, the following are the sequential actions to be taken:

Commence by ascertaining the quantity of calories you presently consume. It is postulated that the typical individual ingests approximately 2000 to 2500 calories per day. Nevertheless, an approximate calculation will prove inadequate and is unlikely to yield the desired outcomes. An accurate numerical value is required for your computations. Fortunately, I have come across a useful online resource that may assist you in completing this task. It is available for your perusal at this location. Utilize it for the purpose of calculating your daily caloric intake and proceed to the subsequent step.

Furthermore, proceed to determine one-fifth of your daily caloric consumption. By utilizing the figure derived from the preceding step, one can ascertain the value equivalent to one-fifth of their daily caloric intake. This is the numerical value that you will utilize throughout your period of fasting.

Once the calculation of the calorie intake for your fasting days has been made, the subsequent task involves the identification of foods that align with that specific calorie count. This step should be straightforward, as conducting a basic online search will yield a plethora of meals accompanied by corresponding recipes that you can utilize.

After completing the aforementioned steps, it is advisable to formulate a comprehensive plan and subsequently commence the immediate execution of this methodology. I would suggest commencing the execution of your proposal at the onset of the week, more specifically on Monday, as this will facilitate the adherence to a more manageable and structured timetable.

In truth, that is the extent of it when it comes to this approach. Now, we shall proceed to examine an alternative approach.

Approach 3: Intermittent Fasting with Controlled Food Consumption

An additional prevailing approach, known for its effectiveness, is commonly referred to as the eat stop eat method. The mentioned program was devised by Brad Pilon, a renowned health and fitness expert who developed it following his graduate studies conducted at the esteemed University of Guelph, located in Canada.

How it works

The operational mechanism is equally straightforward. Based on Brad's perspective, it is advisable to engage in complete fasting for a duration of 24 hours, either once or twice within a seven-day period. An alternative phrasing in a formal tone could be: "To express this idea differently, it is advisable to fast starting from approximately 7 p.m. today and maintain the fast until 7 p.m. tomorrow when transitioning back to your regular eating schedule." It is important to recognize that if you choose to adopt this technique, it is advisable not to exceed fasting more than two times a week. Furthermore, it is imperative that you refrain from fasting on two consecutive days.

For whom is it most suitable?

While the simplicity of this technique may appear evident, not all individuals may adeptly carry it out. This method is well-suited for individuals who lead busy lives and can only allocate one or two days per week to prioritize fasting.

It would be beneficial even for individuals demonstrating sufficient discipline to abstain from food for a duration of 24 hours. As it is apparent to you, this can prove to be a difficult undertaking for the majority of individuals.

How to do it

Do you find yourself persuaded to give this method a try? "If such is the case, here are a few procedural measures you can undertake:

To begin, envision a typical week in your mind. Kindly consider on which day (or possibly two) you anticipate having the highest level of commitments. An eventful day enhances the probability of fasting for a complete twenty-four hours without drawing significant attention to the matter. Additionally, you may opt for a day that is typically less occupied, such as a weekend day.

During the designated period of fasting, it is advisable to plan the consumption of a few non-caloric beverages as a means to alleviate hunger. It is imperative to abstain from consuming any calories throughout the course of this day. This requirement holds significant importance in ensuring the efficacy of this approach. Beverage options include green tea, water, low-calorie soda, or black coffee.

During the usual days of eating, plan and incorporate nourishing, unprocessed meals. Refrain from consuming any unhealthy or processed food items. Also, avoid binge eating. It is advisable to consume food in a manner that reflects the absence of fasting. If one were to engage in excessive consumption of food as a means of compensating for the deficit in caloric intake, it would ultimately nullify the advantageous outcomes associated with the entirety of the program. If you possess uncertainty regarding this matter, it is advisable to adhere to the recommended caloric intake range of 2,000 to 2,500 calories.

Upon further contemplation, implementing this technique may appear akin to a valuable cognitive tool, particularly if one is fully committed to the endeavor. Engaging in intermittent fasting on a weekly basis can appear significantly more manageable compared to adhering to it on alternate days. Hence, if you are seeking to obtain the advantages of intermittent fasting without substantial commitment, this approach may become your preferred choice.

Allow us to transition to a different approach.

www.ingramcontent.com/pod-product-compliance
Lightning Source LLC
Chambersburg PA
CBHW051724020426

42333CB00014B/1146